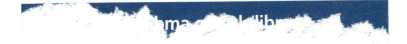

Book 3

MRCP 2

Practice Questions & Answers

Haematology, Neurology, Ophthalmology and Rheumatology

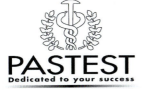

PASTEST
Dedicated to your success

Book 3

MRCP 2

Practice Questions & Answers

Haematology, Neurology, Ophthalmology and Rheumatology

Edited by

Philip Kelly MBBS MRCP
Department of Diabetes and Metabolism
Royal London Hospital
London

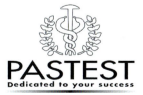

PASTEST
Dedicated to your success

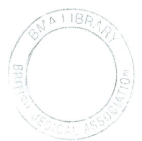

First published 2004

ISBN: 1 904627 27 7

A catalogue record for this book is available from the British Library.

The information contained within this book was obtained by the authors from reliable sources. However, while every effort has been made to ensure its accuracy, no responsibility for loss, damage or injury occasioned to any person acting or refraining from action as a result of information contained herein can be accepted by the publishers or authors.

PasTest Revision Books and Intensive Courses

PasTest has been established in the field of postgraduate medical education since 1972, providing revision books and intensive study courses for doctors preparing for their professional examinations. Books and courses are available for the following specialties:

MRCGP, MRCP Part 1 and 2, MRCPCH Part 1 and 2, MRCPsych, MRCS, MRCOG, DRCOG, DCH, FRCA, PLAB.

For further details contact:

PasTest, Freepost, Knutsford, Cheshire WA16 7BR
Tel: 01565 752000 Fax: 01565 650264
www.pastest.co.uk   enquiries@pastest.co.uk

Text prepared by Vision Typesetting Ltd, Manchester
Printed and bound by Cambrian Printers, Aberystwyth

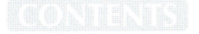

CONTENTS

Haematology
Claire J Hemmaway MRCP MRCPath
Specialist Registrar in Paediatric Haematology, Hammersmith Hospital, London.

Neurology
David L H Bennett MB PhD MRCP
Specialist Registrar in Neurology , Department of Neurology ,
King's College Hospital, London.

Ophthalmology
Jasmin K Singh MBBS MRCOphth
Senior House Officer in Ophthalmology , The Western Eye Hospital, London.

Amir Hamid BMedSci BMBS MRCOphth
Senior House Officer in Ophthalmology , Manchester Royal Eye Hospital, Manchester.

Rheumatology
William G Dixon MRCP
Clinical Research Fellow, **arc** Epidemiology Unit and Specialist Registrar in Rheumatology, University of Manchester, Manchester.

ACKNOWLEDGEMENTS

I would like to express my gratitude to the team at PasTest particularly Cathy Dickens for her unswerving support and tolerance during the preparation of this series. Many patients have been gracious enough to contribute to our ongoing education by allowing their images to be used in these volumes. The series would have been impossible without the help of the following: Mrs Sue Hemmaway for preparation of the haematology section; Dr Philip Beer and David Roper, Hammersmith Hospital, for help with blood films; Dr Mark Layton, Consultant haematologist, Hammersmith Hospital; Mr Riordan-Eva, Consultant ophthalmologist, Kings College Hospital; Medical Photography, Radiology and Medicine at King George Hospital, Ilford; Medical Illustration at Barts and The London School of Medicine and Dentistry; Radiology and The Department of Diabetes and Metabolism at Barts and The London NHS Trust.

Philip Kelly

The MRCP (UK) Part 2 written examination consists of two 3 hour papers, each with up to 100 multiple choice questions; they are either 1 from 5 (best of 5) or 'n' from many, where 2 answers are chosen from 10. Each question will have a clinical scenario and might contain investigations to interpret; many might also contain an image. There is a pass mark agreed by the examiners but a candidate's performance is also assessed in relation to other candidates.

This 3 book series provides practice questions with extensive explanations to aid candidates preparing for the examination. The authors are all clinicians writing sections in their chosen fields and as such have been chosen for their clear understanding of the required knowledge base for this important exam. The breadth of knowledge for this exam is vast and they have attempted to cover the 'syllabus' as completely as possible. Great care has been taken to explain areas that cause difficulty as thoroughly as possible. No apology is made where the format of the questions differs slightly from the exam. These books are not merely practice papers but educational aids and where a topic can be best explained by diversion from the strict format of the exam, for the sake of understanding, this has been done.

This book covers haematology , neurology , ophthalmology and rheumatology and is best taken – in concert with its colleagues within the series – as a supplement to a thorough clinical grounding, the general medical texts and the core clinical journals.

Any comments or suggestions on this book or the series will be gratefully received.

Chapter One

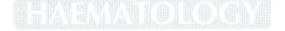

Case 1

A 38-year-old Nigerian lady was referred to the Gastroenterology Clinic for investigation of hyperbilirubinaemia. Her past medical history included a cholecystectomy for gallstone disease more than 10 years ago.

On examination she was jaundiced and pale. There was no lymphadenopathy. A splenic tip was palpable.

Her blood results were as follows:

Hb	8.8 g/dL
Reticulocytes	4% (absolute count 300 × 10^9/L)
WCC	8.9 × 10^9/L
Platelets	156 × 10^9/L
MCV	96 fL
MCH	30 pg
MCHC	37 g/dL
Hb electrophoresis	HbF 0.9% HbA_2 2.8% HbA 96%
U&Es	Normal
Bilirubin	56 μmol/L
ALP	100 U/L
AST	30 U/L
ALT	30 U/L
γGT	32 U/L

1   What are the first three investigations you must do?

☐ A Blood film
☐ B Haptoglobins
☐ C Split bilirubin
☐ D Osmotic fragility
☐ E Heat stability test
☐ F Liver/gallbladder ultrasound
☐ G Direct Coombs' test
☐ H Malaria film
☐ I Glucose-6-phosphate dehydrogenase (G6PD) levels

2   Which three diagnoses are in the differential diagnosis?

☐ A   A membrane disorder, eg hereditary spherocytosis (HS)
☐ B   G6PD deficiency
☐ C   Autoimmune haemolytic anaemia (AIHA)
☐ D   A haemoglobinopathy
☐ E   Haemolytic uraemic syndrome (HUS)
☐ F   Disseminated intravascular coagulation (DIC)
☐ G   Thrombotic thrombocytopenic purpura (TTP)
☐ H   Malaria
☐ I   Paroxysmal nocturnal haemoglobinuria (PNH)
☐ J   Gilbert's syndrome

The film is shown below:

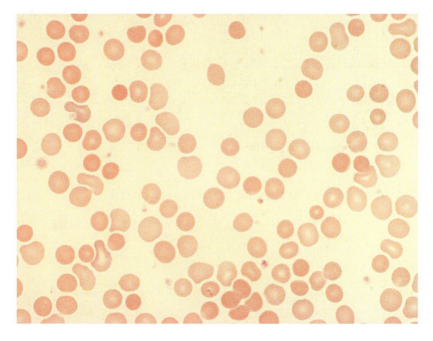

3   What is the diagnosis?

☐ A   A membrane disorder, eg HS   ☐ F   DIC
☐ B   G6PD deficiency   ☐ G   TTP
☐ C   AIHA   ☐ H   Malaria
☐ D   A haemoglobinopathy   ☐ I   PNH
☐ E   HUS   ☐ J   Gilbert's syndrome

Case 2

A 16-year-old Nigerian girl presented to A&E with weakness down the left side of her body. She had been in a lesson at school when the weakness developed suddenly. She was on no medications and had no past medical history apart from mild intermittent joint and bone pains. Her mother had been diagnosed with SLE 5 years earlier. Her father was well and worked in the City as an accountant. She had one sister who was well. She had been born prematurely at 25 weeks.

On examination she was jaundiced and had 4/5 weakness affecting her left upper and left lower limbs. Her face was spared. A systolic murmur was heard at the left sternal edge.

On further questioning, she maintained that her sclera were always yellow.

Her blood test results were as follows:

Hb	8.0 g/dL
MCV	90 fL
WCC	16×10^9/L
Platelets	550×10^9/L
Reticulocytes	5% (absolute count 200×10^9/L)
DCT	Negative
U&Es	Normal
Bilirubin	35 µmol/L
ALP	90 U/L
AST	25 U/L
ALT	30 U/L
LDH	1500 U/L
PT	11 s
APTT	30 s
TT	18 s
Fibrinogen	2.5 g/L

1   Which investigation would you do first?

A Thrombophilia screen

B Magnetic resonance angiography (MRA)

C Lupus anticoagulant

D Autoimmune profile

E Anti cardiolipin antibodies

F Lumbar puncture

G Hb electrophoresis

H Carotid Doppler

I Echocardiogram

J Homocysteine levels

2 How would you manage this patient?

- ☐ A Aspirin
- ☐ B Thrombolytic therapy
- ☐ C Blood transfusion
- ☐ D Exchange blood transfusion
- ☐ E Warfarin
- ☐ F Heparin
- ☐ G Steroids
- ☐ H Carotid endarterectomy
- ☐ I Closure of ventriculo-septal defect

Case 3

A 25-year-old Asian lady presented to her GP again with increasing tiredness, lethargy and easy bruising.

Her blood results were as follows:

Hb	8.2 g/dL
MCV	69 fL
MCH	21 pg
RCC	3.8×10^{12}/L
RDW	24
Platelets	500×10^9/L
WCC	10.9×10^9/L
Neutrophils	7.7×10^9/L

The film is shown below:

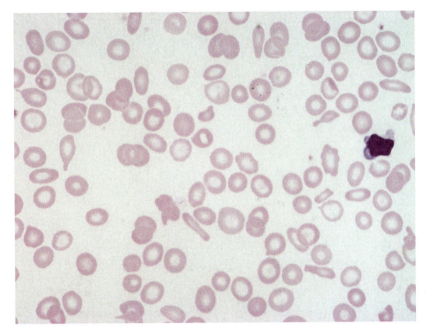

1   What is the diagnosis?

- [ ] A   α-Thalassaemia trait
- [ ] B   β-Thalassaemia trait
- [ ] C   Acute blood loss
- [ ] D   Iron deficiency anaemia
- [ ] E   Acute myeloid leukaemia (AML)

2 What three features shown in the blood film suggest the diagnosis?

- ☐ A Acanthocytes
- ☐ B Pencil cells
- ☐ C A dysplastic neutrophil
- ☐ D Target cells
- ☐ E Macrocytes
- ☐ F Hypochromia
- ☐ G A hyperlobulated neutrophil
- ☐ H Hyperchromia
- ☐ I Microcytosis
- ☐ J Howell–Jolly bodies

Case 4

A 27-year-old Afro-Caribbean man presented to A&E with priapism. Otherwise he felt well in himself. The only other finding on examination was a left upper quadrant mass, which extended 7 cm below the costophrenic angle.

Full blood count results were as follows:

Hb   11 g/dL
WCC 700×10^9/L
Platelets 1400×10^9/L

The film is shown below:

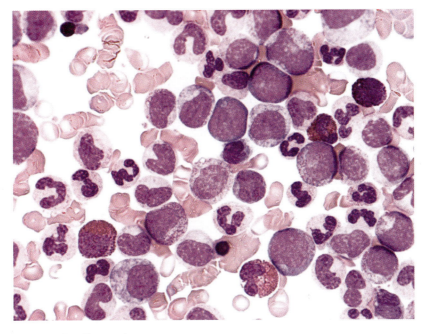

1   What is the diagnosis?

☐ A   Sickle cell disease (SCD)
☐ B   Acute myeloid leukaemia (AML)
☐ C   Chronic myeloid leukaemia (CML)
☐ D   Acute lymphoblastic leukaemia (ALL)
☐ E   Chronic lymphocytic leukaemia (CLL)
☐ F   High-grade non-Hodgkin's lymphoma (NHL)
☐ G   Follicular lymphoma
☐ H   Sildenafil overdose

2   Which cytogenetic abnormality is associated with this disorder?

☐   A   t(4;11)
☐   B   +13
☐   C   +19
☐   D   t(9;22)
☐   E   t(14;18)
☐   F   t(8;14)
☐   G   t(8;21)
☐   H   t(9;11)

Case 5

A 29-year-old Afro-Caribbean man with CML receives a sibling bone marrow transplant.

Seventeen days after the transplant his counts are:

Hb	8.5 g/dL
WCC	0.1×10^9/L
Neutrophils	0.0×10^9/L
Platelets	15×10^9/L
CRP	245 mg/L

He develops fevers of 40 °C, pleuritic chest pain and haemoptysis. He denies shortness of breath at rest or on exertion. His oxygen saturations are 97% on air.

The CXR and CT scan are shown below and on the next page respectively:

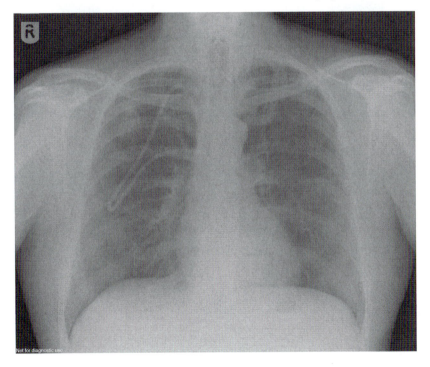

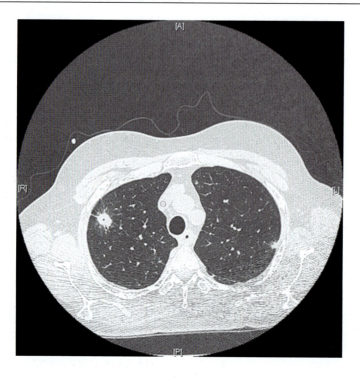

1 What infection would you be most suspicious of with this history and radiological appearance?

☐ A *Pneumocystis* pneumonia (PCP)
☐ B Fungal chest infection
☐ C Cytomegalovirus (CMV) pneumonitis
☐ D Respiratory syncytial (RSV) pneumonitis
☐ E Hospital-acquired bronchopneumonia
☐ F Tuberculosis
☐ G *Staphylococcus aureus* abscess

Case 6

A 65-year-old Moroccan diplomat presented to hospital with a 3-month history of fatigue. He was a heavy drinker but did not smoke. He had travelled widely as part of his job – throughout Africa, Asia, Europe and America. He had a past history of rheumatoid arthritis, treated in the past with steroids, but the disease was currently quiescent. He had had a deep venous thrombosis (DVT) 6 years earlier for which he had been treated with warfarin for 6 months.

On examination he had a low-grade fever, he was pale, jaundiced and had hepatosplenomegaly with the liver being 5 cm below the costal margin and the spleen 17 cm below the costal margin. There was no peripheral lymphadenopathy and no evidence of an active arthropathy.

His blood results are shown below:

Hb	6.7 g/dL
WCC	3.0×10^9/L
Neutrophils	1.9×10^9/L
Lymphocytes	0.7×10^9/L
Platelets	83×10^9/L
Reticulocytes	3.85% (absolute count 250×10^9/L)
Film	Polychromasia
	Target cells
	Spherocytes
	Thrombocytopenia
ESR	132 mm/h
B_{12} and folate	Normal
Serum iron	12 µmol/L
TIBC	40 µmol/L
Ferritin	300 µg/L
Transferrin saturation	10%
DCT positive	IgG 5+, C3D 4+
Haptoglobins	Reduced
U&Es	Normal
Bilirubin	37 µmol/L (conjugated 8 µmol/L)
AST	80 U/L
ALT	60 U/L
ALP	100 U/L
γGT	63 U/L
LDH	530 U/L
Protein electrophoresis	IgM kappa paraprotein 2 g/L
Serum cryoprotein	Not detected

1   What is the main cause of the anaemia?

- ☐ A   Iron deficiency
- ☐ B   Acute blood loss
- ☐ C   Anaemia of chronic disease
- ☐ D   Myelodysplasia
- ☐ E   Non-Hodgkin's lymphoma
- ☐ F   Haemolysis
- ☐ G   Hypersplenism
- ☐ H   None of the above

2   Choose three possible differential diagnoses from the following list:

- ☐ A   Lymphoproliferative disorder
- ☐ B   Chronic liver disease
- ☐ C   Autoimmune haemolytic anaemia
- ☐ D   Acute myeloid leukaemia
- ☐ E   Multiple myeloma
- ☐ F   Chronic myeloid leukaemia
- ☐ G   Myelofibrosis
- ☐ H   Acute hepatitis

Case 7

A 55-year-old man presented to his GP feeling tired, weak and generally unwell. He gave a history of increasing shortness of breath over the last few weeks and a non-productive cough. His past medical history included hypertension, stable angina, diabetes mellitus and rheumatoid arthritis.

On examination, he was pale and had pitting ankle oedema. His BP was 170/100 mmHg. Otherwise, examination was unremarkable.

His bloods counts were as follows:

Hb	6.3 g/dL	ESR	75 mm/h
MCV	89 fL	U&Es	Normal
Platelets	155×10^9/L	LFTs	Normal
WCC	10.2×10^9/L	TSH	0.2 mU/L
Neutrophils	5.6×10^9/L	T_4	9 pmol/L
Reticulocytes	0% (absolute count 0×10^9/L)		

His CXR is shown below:

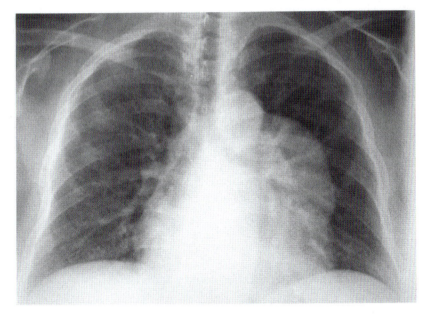

1   **What are the differential diagnoses, based on the CXR alone? (five answers)**

☐   A   Hodgkin's disease
☐   B   Mediastinal non-Hodgkin's lymphoma
☐   C   Lung carcinoma
☐   D   Dissecting thoracic aortic aneurysm
☐   E   Teratoma
☐   F   Sarcoidosis
☐   G   Tuberculosis
☐   H   Pneumonia
☐   I   Thymoma
☐   J   Multiple myeloma
☐   K   Thyroid tumour
☐   L   Syphilitic aortitis

While being investigated for her abnormal CXR she requires a blood transfusion every 3–4 weeks. Her anaemia is investigated:

B_{12}	160 ng/L
Folate	7 µg/L
Ferritin	200 µg/L
Film	Normocytic anaemia with a complete absence of polychromasia

2   **What is the cause of the anaemia?**

☐   A   Myelodysplasia
☐   B   Parvovirus infection
☐   C   Carcinoma of the lung with bone marrow involvement
☐   D   Red cell aplasia
☐   E   Anaemia of chronic disease
☐   F   Mixed haematinic deficiency
☐   G   Acute blood loss

On further questioning this lady also complains of diplopia while reading.

3   **What additional investigation could you perform?**

☐   A   Thyroid autoantibodies
☐   B   LP and cytology
☐   C   Parvovirus titres
☐   D   CT orbit
☐   E   Bronchoscopy
☐   F   Tensilon® test

Case 8

A 60-year-old Nigerian gentleman presents in the UK for a second opinion. Three years before he had been told he was anaemic. He had splenomegaly to below the umbilicus and a liver edge. He had a bone marrow in Nigeria which was inconclusive. His past medical history includes hypertension. He has travelled extensively throughout Africa and has had recurrent attacks of malaria, treated with chloroquine and, most recently, Paludrine®.

He is pale and has splenomegaly as described above. He has no stigmata of liver disease. On auscultation of his heart sounds he has a systolic murmur, loudest at the apex. There is no palpable lymphadenopathy.

His investigation results are shown below:

Hb	5.9 g/dL
MCV	85 fL
MCH	27.4 pg
WCC	6.6×10^9/L
Neutrophils	4.8×10^9/L
Lymphocytes	1.3×10^9/L
Platelets	120×10^9/L
Reticulocytes	3.3% (absolute count 83×10^9/L)
G6PD	205 U/gHb (raised)
Folate	10 µg/L
B_{12}	300 ng/L
Ferritin	706 µg/L
Serum iron	10 µmol/L
TIBC	56 µmol/L
Malaria film	Negative
U&Es	Normal
Bilirubin	26 µmol/L
ALP	100 U/L
ALT	30 U/L
AST	30 U/L
LDH	807 U/L
Uric acid	0.45 mmol/L
Albumin	40 g/L
DCT	Negative
Hep A/B/C serology	Negative (IgG and IgM)
US abdomen	Spleen 21 cm

1   What are the three most likely diagnoses?

- ☐ A   CML
- ☐ B   Amyloidosis
- ☐ C   Chronic liver disease
- ☐ D   Gaucher's disease
- ☐ E   Leishmaniasis
- ☐ F   Myelodysplasia
- ☐ G   Myelofibrosis
- ☐ H   Tropical splenomegaly
- ☐ I   Felty's syndrome
- ☐ J   Sickle cell disease
- ☐ K   AML
- ☐ L   Autoimmune haemolytic anaemia (AIHA)
- ☐ M CLL

2   Which three diagnostic tests would you do to differentiate between your three diagnoses?

- ☐ A   Bone marrow
- ☐ B   Rectal biopsy and stain with Congo red
- ☐ C   Splenic biopsy
- ☐ D   *Leishmania* serology
- ☐ E   Rheumatoid factor
- ☐ F   Malarial antibody titres
- ☐ G   Leucocyte glucocerebrosidase activity
- ☐ H   CT chest/abdomen/pelvis

3   The blood film is shown below: what two features are shown?

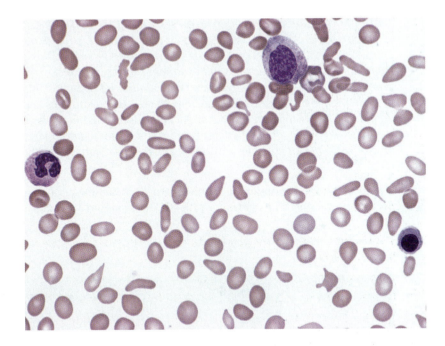

- ☐ A   Tear-drop poikilocytes
- ☐ B   Basophilic stippling
- ☐ C   Hypochromia
- ☐ D   Howell–Jolly bodies
- ☐ E   Heinz bodies
- ☐ F   Polychromasia
- ☐ G   Microcytosis
- ☐ H   Circulating blasts
- ☐ I   Leucoerythroblastic blood film

Case 9

A 51-year-old Caucasian gentleman presented with a flu-like illness and a symmetrical polyarthropathy affecting his knees, ankles, shoulders, elbows and wrists. There was obvious swelling of his knees and ankles and a papular rash over his arms. A full examination was otherwise unremarkable. He was initially treated with antibiotics by his GP but failed to improve. He then presented to A&E with the same symptoms and was admitted for investigation and commenced on anti-inflammatories. X-rays were carried out of all the involved joints, which showed no bony erosions. There was some improvement and he was discharged after a few days.

6 weeks later he was readmitted with shortness of breath, a cough and a persist arthropathy. The rash had resolved. He remained apyrexial.

The CXR is shown below:

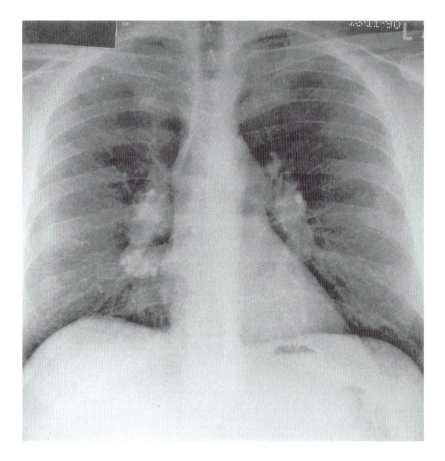

His blood results are shown below:

Hb	15.3 g/dL
WCC	7.0×10^9/L
Platelets	326×10^9/L
MCV	92 fL
ESR	34 mm/h
U&Es	Normal
ALP	90 U/L
AST	40 U/L
ALT	42 U/L
Bilirubin	13 μmol/L
Corrected Ca^{2+}	2.2 mmol/L
Phosphate	0.9 mmol/L
CRP	153 mg/L

Blood gases:

pH	7.4
P_{CO_2}	5.48 kPa
P_{O_2}	9.89 kPa
O_2 saturations	95%

He went on to have a bronchoscopy and lung biopsy which showed non-caseating granulomas and a lymphocytosis (41%) on bronchoalveolar lavage (BAL).

1   What is the most likely diagnosis?

- [ ] A   Tuberculosis
- [ ] B   Teratoma
- [ ] C   Parvovirus infection
- [ ] D   Brucellosis
- [ ] E   Rheumatoid arthritis
- [ ] F   Sarcoidosis
- [ ] G   Hodgkin's disease
- [ ] H   Lung carcinoma
- [ ] I   Cat scratch disease
- [ ] J   Non-Hodgkin's lymphoma
- [ ] K   Polyarteritis nodosa

He is treated for his underlying condition successfully. He continued to be followed up regularly. At one of these routine follow-ups he has the following full blood count:

Hb	18.2 g/dL
RCC	6.4×10^{12}/L
Hct	0.52
MCV	80 fL
WCC	11×10^9/L
Neutrophils	7×10^9/L
Platelets	400×10^9/L
SpO_2	91% on air

2   What is the diagnosis?

- [ ] A   Essential thrombocytosis
- [ ] B   Primary polycythaemia rubra vera
- [ ] C   Secondary polycythaemia
- [ ] D   Reactive thrombocytosis
- [ ] E   Iron deficiency
- [ ] F B_{12} deficiency
- [ ] G   Neutrophilia secondary to steroids
- [ ] H   Dehydration
- [ ] I   Chronic myeloid leukaemia

Case 10

An 80-year-old Indian gentleman, who has been in this country for 30 years but who frequently goes back to India (last visit more than 1 year previously), presented to his GP non-specifically unwell and had a large bruise over his hip following a fall. His past medical history included hypertension, angina and hypercholesterolaemia.

On examination he was apyrexial. His BP was 180/70 mmHg. There were numerous bruises (<2 cm) over his lower limbs and a 10 cm × 10cm bruise over his left hip.

His blood results are shown below:

Hb	10.2 g/dL
MCV	86 fL
WCC	1×10^9/L
Neutrophils	0.02×10^9/L
Lymphocytes	0.2×10^9/L
Platelets	14×10^9/L
Reticulocytes	0.68% (absolute count 21.9×10^9/L)
G6PD activity	Normal
Sodium	134 mmol/L
Potassium	3.9 mmol/L
Urea	9.5 mmol/L
Creatinine	133 μmol/L
Bilirubin	37 μmol/L
ALT	39 U/L
ALP	56 U/L
Bone profile	Normal
CRP	95 mg/L

1   Which three diagnoses are at the top of the differential diagnosis?

- ☐ A   Autoimmune haemolytic anaemia
- ☐ B   Immune thrombocytopenia
- ☐ C   Iron deficiency anaemia
- ☐ D   Non-Hodgkin's lymphoma
- ☐ E   Myelodysplasia
- ☐ F   Chronic lymphocytic leukaemia
- ☐ G   Acute myeloid leukaemia
- ☐ H   Hairy cell leukaemia
- ☐ I   HIV/AIDS

2   The bone marrow is shown below: two diagnoses can be made. What are they?

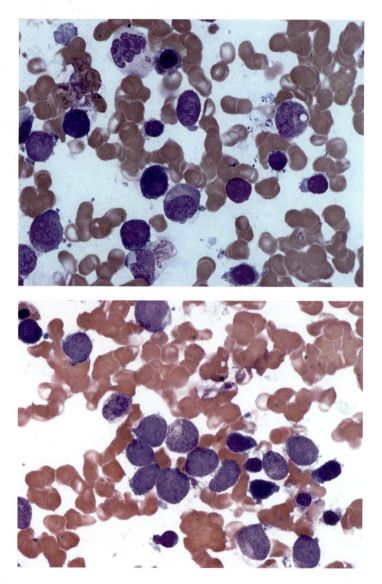

☐   A   Acute myeloid leukaemia   ☐   F   Falciparum malaria
☐   B   Hairy cell leukaemia   ☐   G   Leishmaniasis
☐   C   Chronic lymphocytic leukaemia   ☐   H   Gaucher's disease
☐   D   Non-Hodgkin's lymphoma   ☐   I   Ovale malaria
☐   E   Tuberculosis   ☐   J   Haemophagocytosis

Case 11

A 26-year-old gentleman with sickle cell disease who had recently returned from The Gambia, where he was born, presented to A&E. He complained of abdominal and back pain. His past medical history included recurrent painful crises and two episodes of chest crisis which required ITU admission. He had a cholecystectomy 5 years ago because of recurrent cholecystitis.

He was on hydroxycarbamide (hydroxyurea), 1g daily, which had reduced the frequency of his admissions for painful crises dramatically.

On examination he was pale, pyrexial (38.5 °C), significantly jaundiced and had generalised abdominal tenderness. Chest auscultation was clear. His oxygen saturations were 99% on air.

His blood results are shown below:

Hb	6.0 g/dL
WCC	17×10^9/L
Platelets	500×10^9/L
Neutrophils	15×10^9/L
MCV	112 fL
U&Es	Normal
Bilirubin	78 µmol/L
ALP	110 U/L
AST	26 U/L
ALT	32 U/L
Bone profile	Normal

1   What are the first three investigations you would do?

☐ A   Group and save
☐ B   Haemoglobin S %
☐ C   Chest X-ray
☐ D   Ultrasound (US) of the abdomen
☐ E   Malaria film
☐ F   G6PD levels
☐ G   Blood cultures
☐ H   Urine haemosiderin
☐ I   B$_{12}$ and folate

2   The blood film is shown below. How would you treat this complication? (one answer)

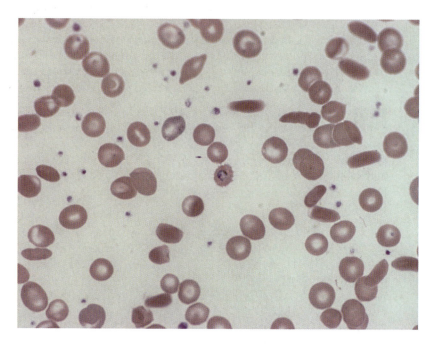

☐ A   Broad-spectrum antibiotics
☐ B   Oxygen
☐ C   Red cell transfusion
☐ D   Analgesia
☐ E   Intravenous fluid
☐ F   Incentive spirometry
☐ G   Physiotherapy
☐ H   None of the above
☐ I   All of the above

3   What investigation should be done prior to commencing therapy?

☐ A   Chest X-ray
☐ B   Blood cultures
☐ C   Haemoglobin S %
☐ D   Ultrasound of the abdomen
☐ E   Reticulocyte count
☐ F   G6PD levels
☐ G   Group and save

Case 12

A 45-year-old Caribbean gentleman was referred to Haematology Outpatients with widespread small-volume lymphadenopathy, night sweats, weight loss and diarrhoea. He admitted to heavy drinking (in excess of 50 units a week) and was a smoker (50 a day). He had had multiple sexual partners in the last 20 years. He had been born in Jamaica, but had lived in the UK for 2 years. He returned to Jamaica frequently.

On examination he had a low-grade pyrexia, widespread small-volume lymphadenopathy, hepatosplenomegaly (liver 2 cm below the costal margin and a splenic tip).

His investigation results were as follows:

Hb	11.6 g/dL
WCC	10.4×10^9/L
Neutrophils	4×10^9/L
Lymphocytes	6×10^9/L
Platelets	140×10^9/L
MCV	94 fL
U&Es	Normal
Bilirubin	18 µmol/L
Albumin	28 mmol/L
ALT	50 U/L
AST	55 U/L
ALP	140 U/L
LDH	900 U/L
Calcium	2.7 mmol/L
Phosphate	0.7 mmol/L
CXR	Normal

1   What is the most likely diagnosis?

- [ ] A   Sarcoidosis
- [ ] B   Tuberculosis
- [ ] C   Human immunodeficiency virus (HIV)
- [ ] D   Adult T-cell leukaemia/lymphoma (ATLL) secondary to HTLV-1 (human T-cell leukaemia virus infection)
- [ ] E   Hodgkin's disease
- [ ] F   Sézary syndrome
- [ ] G   Hyperparathyroidism
- [ ] H   Metastatic carcinoma of the lung

2 He has diarrhoea: what is the cause?

- ☐ A HIV enteropathy
- ☐ B Cytomegalovirus (CMV) enteritis
- ☐ C *Cryptosporidium* infection
- ☐ D *Clostridium difficile* infection
- ☐ E Tuberculous enteritis
- ☐ F *Strongyloides* infection

Case 13

A 54-year-old lady presented to her GP with increased bruising and tiredness. She had been diagnosed with chronic myeloid leukaemia 19 years before. She was initially treated with interferon and then went on to have an autologous bone marrow transplant. She had been completely well for 19 years. Cytogenetic analysis had always shown 0% Philadelphia chromosomes since her transplant.

On examination she had numerous bruises, but there was nothing else to find.

Her blood results showed the following:

Hb	10.2 g/dL	U&Es	Normal
WCC	0.6×10^9/L	Bilirubin	22 μmol/L
Platelets	4×10^9/L	ALT	40 U/L
Neutrophils	0.1×10^9/L	AST	35 U/L
MCV	89 fL	ALP	90 U/L

The film showed thrombocytopenia, leucopenia, a normocytic anaemia and an occasional circulating myeloid precursor.

The bone marrow is shown below:

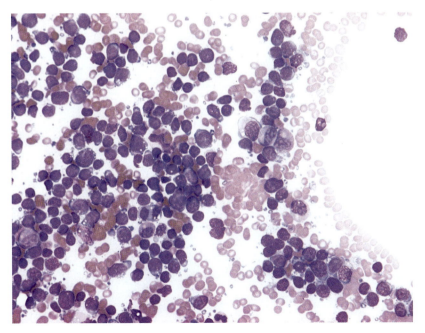

Cytogenetic analysis showed the presence of Philadelphia chromosomes.

1 What is the diagnosis?

- ☐ A Immune thrombocytopenia (ITP)
- ☐ B Myelodysplasia
- ☐ C Chronic myeloid leukaemia (CML) in chronic phase
- ☐ D Chronic myeloid leukaemia (CML) in blast crisis
- ☐ E Acute myeloid leukaemia (AML)
- ☐ F Acute lymphoblastic leukaemia (ALL)

The cells shown in the bone marrow have the following markers on their surface:

CD19 positive	CD7 negative
TDT positive	CD13 negative
CD34 positive	CD33 negative
CD10 positive	CD2 negative
CD79a positive	CD3 negative

2 Which lineage is the current problem in?

- ☐ A B lymphoid
- ☐ B Myeloid
- ☐ C T lymphoid
- ☐ D None of the above

Case 14

A 32-year-old lady presented to A&E with bleeding per vaginam. She is 20 weeks pregnant. On ultrasound there is intrauterine growth retardation (IUGR). She had a DVT aged 30 following a road traffic accident when she fractured her left femur.

Her blood results were as follows:

Hb	10.5 g/dL
WCC	11×10^9/L
Platelets	51×10^9/L
MCV	78 fL
PT	15 s
APTT	58 s
50:50 mix	58 s
TT	12 s
Fibrinogen	2.5 g/dL

1   Which three investigations would you request next to investigate the abnormal blood results?

☐   A   Factor VIII levels
☐   B   Lupus anticoagulant and anti cardiolipin antibodies
☐   C B_{12} and folate
☐   D   Bone marrow
☐   E   Urate
☐   F   Blood pressure
☐   G   Blood film
☐   H   Dipstix urinalysis
☐   I   von Willebrand factor level
☐   J   Haemolysis screen
☐   K   All of the above
☐   L   None of the above

2   What other history would you like to know? (one answer)

- [ ] A   Past obstetric history
- [ ] B   Family history of thrombotic episodes
- [ ] C   Bleeding history
- [ ] D   Family history of early pregnancy loss
- [ ] E   Family history of thrombocytopenia
- [ ] F   Weight loss
- [ ] G   Night sweats
- [ ] H   Warfarin-induced skin necrosis

3   What diagnosis would you consider?

- [ ] A   Acquired haemophilia A
- [ ] B   von Willebrand's disease
- [ ] C   Immune thrombocytopenia
- [ ] D   Antiphospholipid syndrome
- [ ] E   Thrombotic thrombocytopenic purpura

Case 15

A 25-year-old lady who is 34 weeks pregnant (para 2) presented to A&E with a 4-day history of jaundice, easy bruising and a severe headache. There had been no prior problems in the pregnancy.

On examination she was jaundiced. Her BP was 110/75 mmHg. Her temperature was 37 °C. She had several small bruises over her abdomen and legs. Urinanalysis showed protein +++ and blood +++.

Her blood results were as follows:

Hb	8.6 g/dL
WCC	5.6×10^9/L
Neutrophils	4.0×10^9/L
Platelets	7×10^9/L
MCV	90 fL
Reticulocytes	4% (absolute count 200×10^9/L)
U&Es	Normal
Bilirubin	155 μmol/L
AST	25 U/L
ALT	25 U/L
ALP	95 U/L
LDH	5000 U/L
Clotting and fibrinogen	Normal

The film is shown below:

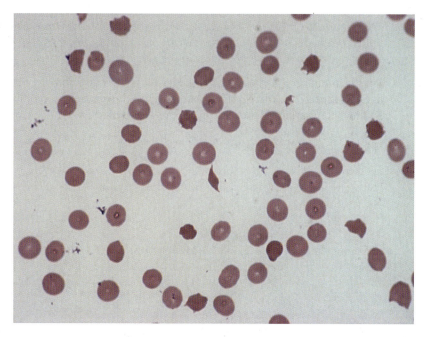

1   What is the most likely diagnosis?

☐ A   Thrombotic thrombocytopenic purpura (TTP)
☐ B   Haemolytic uraemic syndrome (HUS)
☐ C   HELLP syndrome
☐ D   Pre-eclampsia
☐ E   Immune thrombocytopenia

2   What is the correct, evidence-based management?

☐ A   Folic acid
☐ B   Plasma exchange
☐ C   Dialysis
☐ D   Steroids
☐ E   Liver biopsy
☐ F   Intravenous immunoglobulin (IVIG)
☐ G   Bed rest
☐ H   Emergency Caesarean section
☐ I   None of the above

Case 16

A 76-year-old Polish gentleman presented to A&E with a 3-week history of lethargy, shortness of breath, confusion and being 'off his legs'.

On examination he had a chaotic pulse of 140 bpm. His BP was 130/85 mmHg and his SaO_2 99% on air. He was jaundiced and had bibasal inspiratory crepitations on auscultation of his chest. It was impossible to do a full neurological examination on him because he spoke no English and was confused.

His bloods results are shown below:

Hb	5.9 g/dL
WCC	4.0×10^9/L
Neutrophils	2.8×10^9/L
MCV	129 fL
Platelets	90×10^9/L
Reticulocytes	0.5% (absolute count 25×10^9/L)
DCT	Negative
Clotting and fibrinogen	Normal
U&Es	Normal
Bilirubin	50 µmol/L
AST	35 U/L
ALT	35 U/L
ALP	100 U/L
LDH	2500 U/L
T_4	9 pmol/L
TSH	0.2 mU/L

The film is shown below:

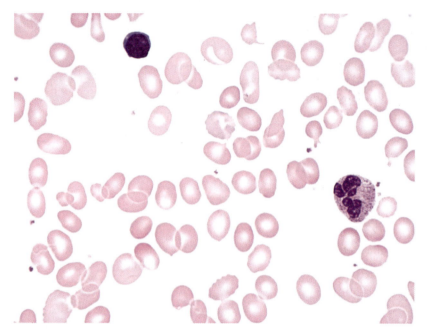

1   What are the two differential diagnoses?

- ☐ A   B$_{12}$ or folate deficiency
- ☐ B   Thrombotic thrombocytopenic purpura
- ☐ C   Immune thrombocytopenic purpura
- ☐ D   High-grade non-Hodgkin's lymphoma
- ☐ E   Hypothyroidism
- ☐ F   Hepatitis
- ☐ G   Myelodysplasia
- ☐ H   Autoimmune haemolytic anaemia

2   What would your next investigation be?

- ☐ A   B$_{12}$ and folate measurements
- ☐ B   Bone marrow
- ☐ C   Bone marrow chromosome analysis
- ☐ D   TSH test
- ☐ E   CT chest/abdomen/pelvis
- ☐ F   Haptoglobins

3   Which two are the correct management?

- ☐ A B_{12} replacement
- ☐ B   Blood transfusion
- ☐ C   Chemotherapy
- ☐ D   Digoxin
- ☐ E   Plasma exchange
- ☐ F   Thyroxine

Case 17

A 60-year-old man is admitted via his GP to your care with streptococcal pneumonia and is treated appropriately. He is a smoker, drinks a bottle of vodka per week and works in a fish market during the week. 10 days after his admission his haemoglobin drops to 9 g/dL from 12 g/dL on admission and he becomes jaundiced. He had been started on ibuprofen for generalised aches and pains.

The next day the blood results were as follows:

Hb	6.4 g/dL
MCV	99 fL
WCC	14.6×10^9/L
Neutrophils	11×10^9/L
Platelets	140×10^9/L
Reticulocytes	6% (absolute count 300×10^9/L)

The film is shown below:

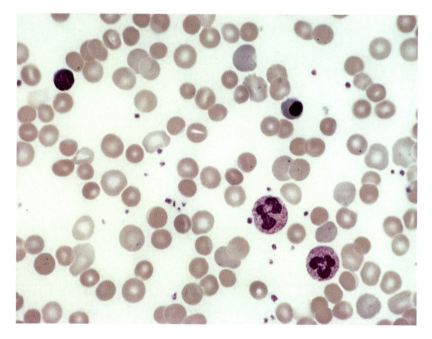

1 Which two investigations would you do next?

- A B_{12} measurement
- B Direct Coombs' test (DCT)
- C LDH
- D Ferritin
- E Oesophagogastroduodenoscopy
- F Folate
- G Colonoscopy
- H None of the above

2 What is the diagnosis?

- A Delayed transfusion reaction
- B Immune haemolytic anaemia
- C Gastrointestinal bleed
- D Iron deficiency
- E Folate deficiency
- F B_{12} deficiency

3 What is implicated in the aetiology of the above diagnosis?

- A A blood transfusion
- B Ibuprofen
- C Folate
- D Peptic ulceration
- E Antibiotic treatment

Case 18

A 60-year-old gentleman presented to his GP with increasing tiredness, shortness of breath and worsening of his angina over the last 10 days.

On examination he was mildly jaundiced and pale. He had no palpable lymphadenopathy or organomegaly. Chest auscultation revealed no abnormality. On auscultation of his heart he had a pansystolic murmur, loudest at the apex.

His blood results were as follows:

Hb   5.1 g/dL
MCV   101 fL
WCC 140×10^9/L
Platelets 200×10^9/L
Reticulocytes 6.2% (absolute count 350×10^9/L)

His blood film is shown below at low power and opposite at high power:

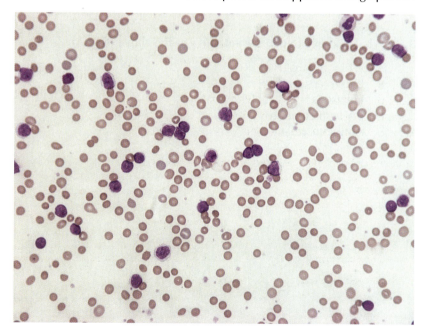

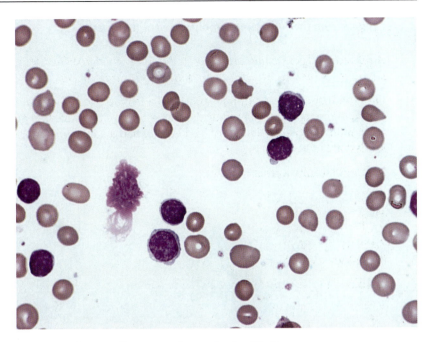

1   What are the two diagnoses shown in the film?

☐   A   Hodgkin's disease
☐   B   Diffuse large B-cell lymphoma
☐   C   Chronic myeloid leukaemia (CML)
☐   D   Autoimmune haemolytic anaemia (AIHI)
☐   E   Iron deficiency
☐   F   Chronic lymphocytic leukaemia (CLL)
☐   G   Sézary syndrome
☐   H B_{12} deficiency
☐   I   Myelofibrosis
☐   J   Acute lymphoblastic leukaemia (ALL)

The following are options to treat the two conditions:

1 Oral chemotherapy
2 B_{12}
3 Ferrous sulphate
4 High-dose steroids
5 Intravenous chemotherapy
6 Radiotherapy
7 Splenectomy
8 Folic acid
9 Blood transfusion.

2   Choose from the following combinations of treatment:

- ☐   A   7 and 8
- ☐   B   1, 4, 8 and 9
- ☐   C   5 and 6
- ☐   D   8 and 9
- ☐   E   4 and 8
- ☐   F   2 and 3 and 4
- ☐   G   None of the above

Case 19

A 33-year-old man is referred to you by his GP with shortness of breath and tiredness. He has hereditary spherocytosis. Eight days prior to the onset of symptoms he had a mild febrile illness, as did his 4-year-old son.

On examination he is pale, jaundiced and a splenic tip is palpable.

Investigations reveal:

Hb	4.5 g/dL
MCV	90 fL
Platelets	160×10^9/L
WCC	10×10^9/L
Lymphocytes	70%
Reticulocytes	0.1% (absolute count 5×10^9/L)
Film	Occasional atypical lymphocytes,
Bilirubin	26 µmol/L
U&Es and LFTs	Normal

1   What is the most likely diagnosis?

☐ A Folic acid deficiency
☐ B B_{12} deficiency
☐ C Large gastrointestinal bleed
☐ D Parvovirus-induced red cell aplasia
☐ E Hypersplenism
☐ F Acute haemolysis
☐ G Epstein–Barr virus infection
☐ H Cytomegalovirus infection

This patient had required a cholecystectomy at the age of 25.

2   What condition could exacerbate the propensity to gallstone formation?

☐ A Gilbert's syndrome
☐ B B_{12} deficiency
☐ C Folate dependency
☐ D Iron deficiency
☐ E Acute bleed
☐ F High-fat diet

Case 20

An Asian lady with recurrent iron deficiency has the following clotting profile:

PT	12.5 s
APPT	44 s
TT	15 s (10–15 s)
Fibrinogen	5.2 g/L
Bleeding time	11 min
Factor VIII level	30 U/dL

1   What is the possible diagnosis, to explain her recurrent anaemia?

A   Vitamin K deficiency
B   Haemophilia A
C   von Willebrand's disease
D   Warfarin overdose
E   Amyloidosis
F   Hyperfibrinogenaemia
G   Hypofibrinogenaemia
H   Ehlers–Danlos syndrome
I   Systemic lupus erythematosus (SLE)
J   Haemophilia B
K   Factor XI deficiency

Chapter Two

NEUROLOGY

Case 1

A 28-year-old man presents to A&E complaining of difficulty swallowing, dry mouth, altered speech and double vision over the last 5 days, and today he had difficulty walking. He has a 10-year history of intravenous heroin use.

On examination he is apyrexial, he has a bilateral ptosis, reduced abduction of both eyes and his pupils are not reactive to light. He has bilateral facial weakness, he is dysarthric and his cough is bovine. Examination of his limbs shows that he is generally thin, there are multiple marks from injection sites, he has a proximal weakness in the upper and lower limbs, his reflexes are reduced but present, plantar reflexes are flexor, sensory examination is normal. His respiratory rate is 20/min; oxygen saturation is 96% on air; forced vital capacity is 900 mL.

Creatine kinase (CK)   190 U/L

1 What is the diagnosis?

- A Guillain–Barré syndrome
- B Myasthenia gravis
- C Polio
- D Wound botulism
- E Drug-induced myopathy

2 Your next management step is to:

- A Give botulinum antitoxin and penicillin
- B Give pyridostigmine
- C Give intravenous immunoglobulin
- D Get urgent anaesthetic review for transfer to ITU
- E Transfer to a neurology centre for plasma exchange

Case 2

You are referred a 70-year-old right-handed man in the Rapid-Access Stroke Clinic. He describes an episode which occurred 2 months ago. He was eating and developed acute-onset weakness and numbness of his left arm. This lasted 5 minutes and then completely resolved. He is hypertensive and smokes 10 cigarettes a day. His current medication is aspirin 75 mg and ramipril 5 mg.

On examination his blood pressure is 130/86 mmHg, a carotid bruit is heard on the right, neurological examination is normal.

He has had a number of investigations:

FBC	Normal
Renal function	Normal
Fasting glucose	3.9 mmol/L
Fasting cholesterol	5.0 mmol/L
ECG	Normal sinus rhythm
Echocardiogram	Left ventricular hypertrophy
Carotid Doppler	55% stenosis of the right carotid artery

1   The appropriate management is to:

- ☐ A   Increase the dose of aspirin
- ☐ B   Add dipyridamole to aspirin
- ☐ C   Replace aspirin with clopidogrel and simvastatin
- ☐ D   Add dipyridamole and simvastatin
- ☐ E   Add dipyridamole and refer the patient for carotid endarterectomy

Case 3

A 20-year-old man is admitted with a flare of his ulcerative colitis and treated with intravenous hydrocortisone. About 24 hours following admission he becomes increasingly drowsy. His Glasgow Coma Scale (GCS) score drops to 8 and his temperature is 37.5 °C, he has bilateral papilloedema, he is flexing all his limbs to painful stimuli, all his tendon reflexes are present and symmetrical and both plantar reflexes are extensor. He subsequently has a generalised seizure and is intubated and ventilated.

His blood tests are:

Sodium	148 mmol/L
Potassium	3.1 mmol/L
Urea	10.4 mmol/L
Creatinine	120 µmol/L
Hb	10.1 g/dL
MCV	79 fL
WCC	16.5×10^9/L
Platelets	430×10^9/L
ESR	80 mm/h

His CT head with contrast is shown below:

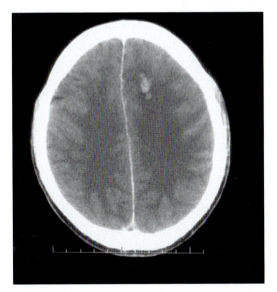

1 What is the diagnosis?

- ☐ A Sagittal sinus thrombosis
- ☐ B Bacterial meningitis
- ☐ C Intracerebral abscess
- ☐ D Intracerebral haemorrhage
- ☐ E Cerebral oedema

2 The correct treatment is:

- ☐ A Intravenous ceftriaxone
- ☐ B Therapeutic anticoagulation with heparin
- ☐ C Intravenous dexamethasone
- ☐ D Referral to Neurosurgery Department for evacuation of clot
- ☐ E Rehydration with normal saline

Case 4

A 30-year-old right-handed man attends A&E. Yesterday he went mountain biking. Today he noticed a pain in his neck and his left arm feels funny.

On examination he has a right partial ptosis and the right pupil is smaller than the left. The remainder of the cranial nerves are normal. You note slight loss of dexterity in the left hand; there is no weakness or ataxia. His reflexes are brisker on the left than on the right, both plantar reflexes are flexor. He has evidence of sensory neglect in the left upper and left lower limbs.

He has had a CT head which is reported as normal.

1   The best diagnosis is:

- [ ] A   Vertebral artery dissection
- [ ] B   Acute cervical disc protrusion
- [ ] C   Right carotid artery dissection
- [ ] D   Right middle cerebral artery infarct
- [ ] E   Right lateral medullary syndrome

2   The most appropriate next investigation is:

- [ ] A   CT cervical spine
- [ ] B   MRI brain and cervical spine
- [ ] C   Percutaneous angiography
- [ ] D   Plain X-ray of neck
- [ ] E   Carotid Doppler

3   The most appropriate management is:

- [ ] A   Aspirin 300 mg stat
- [ ] B   Thrombolysis with tPA
- [ ] C   Therapeutic anticoagulation with heparin
- [ ] D   Referral to a neurosurgeon
- [ ] E   Analgesia and physiotherapy

Case 5

A 30-year-old lady is brought to hospital by ambulance. The night before, she had complained of nausea and headache to her husband. She had gone to bed and on waking he found that she was confused and irritable.

On admission she was 37.5 °C; GCS was 8; there was neck stiffness; the pupils were equal and reactive; there was no papilloedema or haemorrhages; she flexed all four limbs to pain; the reflexes were brisk throughout; and the plantar reflexes were extensor.

The patient is intubated and ventilated and a CT scan (without contrast) is shown.

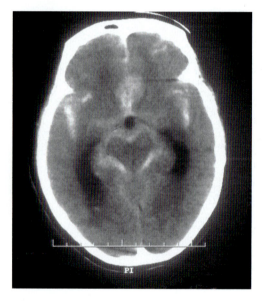

1   The diagnosis is:

- [ ] A   Bacterial meningitis
- [ ] B   Venous sinus thrombosis
- [ ] C   Subarachnoid haemorrhage
- [ ] D   Intracerebral haemorrhage
- [ ] E   Subdural haemorrhage

2   What complication has occurred?

- [ ] A   Abscess formation
- [ ] B   Hydrocephalus
- [ ] C   Middle cerebral artery (MCA) vasospasm
- [ ] D   Malignant MCA syndrome
- [ ] E   Venous infarction

Case 6

A 55-year-old Indian lady attends Outpatients complaining of fatigue and muscle pains, particularly affecting her shoulders and thigh muscles. She has difficulty walking upstairs and difficulty rising from a chair. There is no family history of neuromuscular disorders.

On examination, temporal arteries are normal and non-tender; she has normal cranial nerve examination; she has a proximal weakness in both upper and lower limbs and difficulty rising from a squat. Reflexes and sensory examination are normal.

The GP has helpfully performed a number of blood tests:

Hb	11.0 g/dL
MCV	95 fL
WCC	5.2×10^9/L
Platelets	420×10^9/L
Sodium	140 mmol/L
Potassium	3.6 mmol/L
Urea	7.0 mmol/L
Creatinine	62 µmol/L
Albumin	37 g/L
ALT	20 U/L
ALP	388 U/L
Bilirubin	20 µmol/L
Calcium	2.10 mmol/L
Phosphate	0.8 mmol/L
Creatine kinase	305 U/L

1   The diagnosis is:

- ☐ A   Polymyositis
- ☐ B   Polymyalgia rheumatica
- ☐ C   Myasthenia gravis
- ☐ D   Osteomalacia
- ☐ E   Hypothyroidism

Case 7

A 25-year-old Peruvian man, who came to this country a year ago, is referred to you in A&E. He describes abnormal movements of his left arm. These occur without warning: he describes the arm as stiffening and then shaking for 1 to 5 minutes. He is unable to control the arm during the episode and it often feels weak for 30 minutes to an hour afterwards. He does not have any impairment of consciousness during this period. These episodes are occurring approximately once a week and he had a further episode this morning. His GP has started him on carbamazepine.

He complains of painful thigh muscles and on palpation they are tender; otherwise neurological examination is normal. He is afebrile.

He has had a CT scan which is shown below:

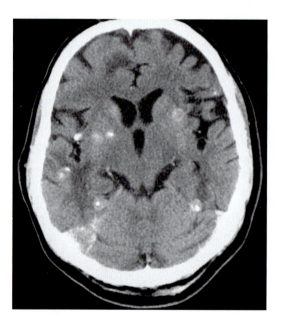

Carbamazepine trough level 22 μmol/L

1   The diagnosis is:

- [ ] A   Neurocysticercosis
- [ ] B   Multiple cerebral metastases
- [ ] C   Cerebral toxoplasmosis
- [ ] D   Cerebral lymphoma
- [ ] E   *Ascaris lumbricoides*

2   Regarding management of his seizures, you would suggest:

☐   A   Increasing carbamazepine and re-checking levels in a week's time
☐   B   Give a loading dose of intravenous phenytoin in A&E
☐   C   Adding sodium valproate to carbamazepine
☐   D   Stopping carbamazepine and substitute phenytoin
☐   E   Giving a stat dose of oral diazepam

Case 8

You are asked to review a patient on the ward. He is 35 years old and drinks 80 units of alcohol a week. He was admitted 2 days ago with vomiting and generalised tonic-clonic seizures. He was treated with thiamine, fluid replacement, diazepam and phenytoin. He is now seizure-free but now complains that he can no longer walk.

On examination he has numerous spider naevi, pupils are equal and reactive and fundoscopy is normal. He has gaze-evoked horizontal nystagmus with reduced eye abduction bilaterally. His speech is slurred but he is lucid and orientated. He has bilateral facial weakness and marked weakness of both upper and lower limbs. His deep tendon reflexes are depressed throughout and both plantar reflexes are extensor.

You review the current blood tests and those performed on admission:

	Admission	Current
Sodium	114	139 mmol/L
Potassium	3.3	4.2 mmol/L
Urea	9.0	5.2 mmol/L
Creatinine	100	80 µmol/L
Albumin	35	35 g/L
ALT	40	42 U/L
ALP	210	200 U/L
γGT	400	390 U/L
Bilirubin	25	24 µmol/L
Calcium	2.30	2.3 mmol/L
Phosphate	0.9	0.9 mmol/L

You request a CT brain which is normal.

1   The diagnosis is:

- ☐ A   Guillain–Barré syndrome
- ☐ B   Brainstem stroke
- ☐ C   Wernicke's encephalopathy
- ☐ D   Central pontine myelinolysis
- ☐ E   Hepatic encephalopathy

Case 9

A 50-year-old man is referred to the clinic because of unsteadiness on walking. He has also had a number of falls. He first noticed his symptoms 3 months ago and they have been getting progressively worse; more recently his speech has become slurred. He has a past history of hypertension which is treated with bendroflumethiazide (bendrofluazide) and he smokes 10 cigarettes a day. He drinks 20 units of alcohol a week.

On examination he has sustained horizontal nystagmus in both directions. He is dysarthric and has marked upper and lower limb ataxia bilaterally. Power is normal throughout, and the sensory examination is also normal.

Routine blood tests, including liver function and thyroid function tests are normal. He has had an MRI brain which is reported as normal with no evidence of cerebellar atrophy.

A lumbar puncture is performed:

CSF glucose	4.0 mmol/L (serum 6.0 mmol/L)
CSF protein	0.8 g/dL
CSF red cell count	5/mm³
CSF white cell count	1 lymphocyte/mm³

Matched oligoclonal bands are positive in CSF and serum.

1   The most likely diagnosis is:

- ☐ A   Alcohol-related cerebellar degeneration
- ☐ B   Multiple sclerosis (MS)
- ☐ C   Friedreich's ataxia
- ☐ D   Paraneoplastic cerebellar degeneration
- ☐ E   Herpes zoster cerebellitis

Case 10

A 60-year-old right-handed lady complains of severe pain in her right shoulder that started 3 weeks ago. This started 1 week after receiving pneumococcal vaccine, which was administered into her right arm. There was no history of trauma. More recently her pain has improved; however she has noted that she is unable to lift her arm above her head.

On examination there is wasting of the deltoid, which is weak, as is the biceps muscle. The right biceps and supinator jerks are absent; the remainder of the reflexes are normal. On sensory examination she has reduced sensation to pinprick over the right shoulder and the lateral aspect of the arm. Examination of the lower limbs is normal.

1   The most likely diagnosis is:

- ☐ A   Axillary nerve palsy
- ☐ B   Cervical disc causing root compression at C7
- ☐ C   Neuralgic amyotrophy
- ☐ D   Neoplastic infiltration of the brachial plexus
- ☐ E   Avulsion injury of the brachial plexus

Case 11

An 18-year-old girl complains of unusual episodes of collapse. Typically these occur when she laughs. She suddenly feels weak as if she has no power in her legs and drops to the ground. She is completely alert and orientated during this time and makes a rapid recovery. She also describes an unusual experience in the morning of waking and not being able to move. She is anxious about her symptoms; she has not been sleeping well at night and feels tired.

Cardiovascular and neurological examinations are normal.

1   The diagnosis is:

- ☐ A   Narcolepsy
- ☐ B   Non-epileptic attack disorder
- ☐ C   Temporal lobe epilepsy
- ☐ D   Hypoglycaemia
- ☐ E   Hypothyroidism

Case 12

A 60-year-old man complains of progressive difficulty with walking over the last 3 months and, more recently, a dry mouth, difficulty swallowing and difficulty passing urine.

On examination he is generally thin; there are no fasciculations. He has clubbing and a fatiguable proximal weakness in both upper and lower limbs. His tendon reflexes are present but depressed, plantar reflexes are flexor. Sensory examination and co-ordination are normal.

A number of blood tests are performed:

Hb	10.5 g/dL
MCV	95 fL
WCC	5.2×10^9/L
Platelets	420×10^9/L
Sodium	141 mmol/L
Potassium	3.8 mmol/L
Creatinine	62 µmol/L
ESR	40 mm/h
Creatine kinase	190 U/L
Anti-ACh receptor Ab Negative	

1   The diagnosis is:

- ☐ A   Polymyositis
- ☐ B   Motor neurone disease
- ☐ C   Myasthenia gravis
- ☐ D   Lambert–Eaton myasthenic syndrome
- ☐ E   Cervical spondylosis

Case 13

A 20-year-old right-handed lady is referred by her GP with unusual episodes. These have occurred since the age of 18 but have recently become more frequent; the last was a week ago. They usually begin with a strange epigastric sensation which rises up. She feels fearful and distant from her surroundings. Her husband describes her as being distant and says that she sometimes picks at objects around her (there may also be chewing movements). She is aware of her heart beating strongly. These episodes last for up to 10 minutes, although she may be confused for up to an hour afterwards. She had one febrile convulsion as a child.

Neurological and cardiovascular examination is normal.

An EEG is performed which is normal and a CT head is normal.

1   The most likely diagnosis is:

☐   A   Panic disorder
☐   B   Phaeochromocytoma
☐   C   Temporal lobe epilepsy
☐   D   Absence seizures
☐   E   Cardiac arrhythmia

2   What should the patient be told about driving?

☐   A   She did not lose consciousness and so can continue to drive
☐   B   She should not drive for 6 months from her last episode
☐   C   You advise her not to drive and that she should inform the DVLA
☐   D   You will inform the DVLA of these episodes
☐   E   She can continue to drive until investigations are complete

Case 14

A 40-year-old man attends A&E. He complains of progressive weakness, paraesthesiae and numbness that began in his feet, spreading up both legs and then involved both his hands over 3 days, associated with fever. Today he has had difficulty passing urine. He has a past history of intravenous heroin use.

On examination he is unkempt, he has multiple injection sites, he has a temperature of 38 °C and a soft systolic murmur is heard at the apex. He is alert and orientated. He complains of pain on passive neck movement and neck stiffness is noted. He has a severe flaccid weakness of both upper and lower limbs and his tendon reflexes are absent. Plantar reflexes are extensor. He complains of reduced sensation to pinprick in the lower and upper limbs, and up to just below the level of the clavicle bilaterally and to the same level on the posterior chest wall. Vibration sense and joint-position sense are also reduced in this distribution.

An urgent MRI cervical spine is performed.

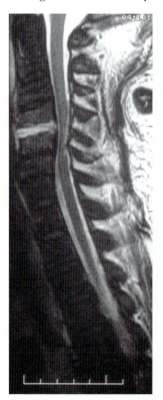

1   The most likely diagnosis is:

☐ A   Anterior spinal artery infarction
☐ B   Transverse myelitis
☐ C   Cervical disc prolapse
☐ D   Spinal abscess
☐ E   Vertebral metastatic deposit

You organise basic blood tests, a septic screen, ECG and chest X-ray.

2   Your next management step should be:

☐ A   Antituberculous treatment
☐ B   Intravenous immunoglobulin treatment
☐ C   Broad-spectrum antibiotics and intravascular dexamethasone
☐ D   Broad-spectrum antibiotics and neurosurgical referral
☐ E   HIV testing

Case 15

A 50-year-old Italian man developed a left foot drop 2 months ago and then 2 weeks ago noted reduced grip strength in his right hand associated with pain in the fingers. He describes a fleeting rash on his feet. He has chronic hepatitis C. His current medication is bendroflumethiazide (bendrofluazide) 2.5 mg.

On examination he has weakness of the right first dorsal interosseus and abductor digiti minimi, as well as ankle dorsiflexion and eversion on the left. There is a patch of reduced sensation to pinprick on the dorsum of the left foot and on the right little finger and ring finger. Vibration sense and proprioception are preserved. Reflexes are all present.

Urinalysis reveals protein +, blood ++ and no bilirubin. A number of blood tests are performed:

Hb	11.6 g/dL
MCV	95 fL
WCC	5.2×10^9/L
Platelets	420×10^9/L
Sodium	142 mmol/L
Potassium	3.9 mmol/L
Creatinine	150 µmol/L
ESR	50 mm/h
Creatine kinase	180 U/L
Albumin	33 g/L
ALT	160 U/L
ALP	150 U/L
γGT	200 U/L
Bilirubin	24 µmol/L
ANA	Negative
ANCA	Negative
Prothrombin time	17 s
Plasma glucose	5.4 mmol/L
CRP	40 mg/L

1 What is the pattern of the neuropathy?

☐ A Generalised sensorimotor neuropathy
☐ B Right radial, left common peroneal
☐ C Right ulnar, left tibial
☐ D Right median, left sciatic
☐ E Right ulnar, left common peroneal

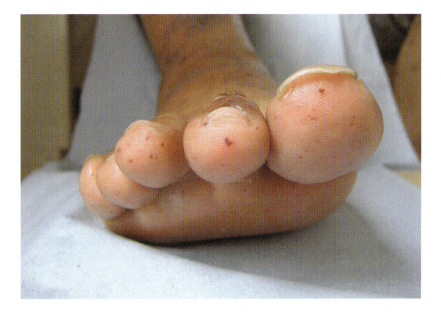

2   The most likely diagnosis is:

☐   A   Vitamin B$_{12}$ deficiency
☐   B   Chronic inflammatory demyelinating polyneuropathy (CIDP)
☐   C   Cryoglobulinaemia
☐   D   Paraneoplastic neuropathy
☐   E   Wegener's granulomatosis

Case 16

A 65-year-old man was diagnosed with idiopathic Parkinson's disease 5 years ago when he developed a rest tremor and stiffness of the left arm. He was commenced on levodopa therapy 3 years ago when his walking slowed and he says this was helpful. He was admitted to hospital after having a fall and fracturing his hip. This was successfully repaired but the physiotherapists feel that he is much slower to mobilise than they would expect. His current medication is co-careldopa 125 mg qds, tramadol 50 mg bd and metoclopramide 10 mg tds.

On examination he has poverty of facial expression, his speech is soft and he has difficulty swallowing. He has marked rigidity in all four limbs a rest tremor, more marked in the left arm, and is very bradykinetic. He is able to stand with difficulty but cannot walk. He has been noted to have a labile blood pressure since admission.

1   You should:

- ☐ A   Gradually increase levodopa dose
- ☐ B   Perform a full septic screen
- ☐ C   Add an anticholinergic agent such as trihexyphenidyl (benzhexol)
- ☐ D   Change metoclopramide to domperidone
- ☐ E   Inform the patient that he has multiple systems atrophy

Case 17

An 80-year-old man is admitted from a nursing home. He has a 3-day history of headache and today has become increasingly confused.

On examination he has a temperature of 38 °C and has neck stiffness. He has a GCS of 12 on admission and has a witnessed generalised tonic-clonic seizure.

A CT is performed which is normal. A lumbar puncture is performed. The opening pressure is 24 cmH$_2$O and the CSF is cloudy:

CSF glucose	3.5 mmol/L
CSF protein	0.8 g/dL
CSF red cell count	50/mm^3
CSF white cell count	75 lymphocytes, 5 polymorphs/mm^3
Gram stain	Gram-positive rods
Serum glucose	6.0 mmol/L

1   The treatment of choice is:

☐ A Benzylpenicillin
☐ B Ceftriaxone and clarithromycin
☐ C Ceftriaxone and ampicillin
☐ D Aciclovir
☐ E Antituberculous therapy

Case 18

The photograph shows the eyes of a 60-year-old man who developed diplopia, a complete left ptosis over a number of days and then a right hemiparesis.

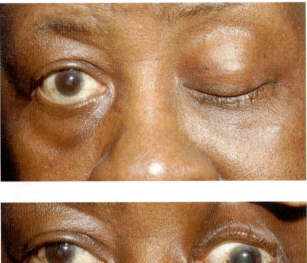

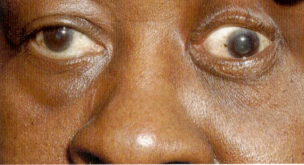

1   Where is the lesion?

- [ ] A   Left internal capsule
- [ ] B   Left frontal lobe
- [ ] C   Left cerebellopontine angle
- [ ] D   Left orbit
- [ ] E   Left midbrain

Case 19

A 50-year-old man who lives alone is found collapsed at home; he is in respiratory failure and is intubated by paramedics. His admission bloods are shown below. On ITU he is treated for pneumonia but when his sedation is reduced he is noted to have facial and limb weakness and he is difficult to wean off the ventilator. Neurophysiology is performed on ITU and the figure shows the results of repetitive nerve stimulation.

Hb	13.8 g/dL
WCC	9.3×10^9/L
MCV	99 fL
Platelets	129×10^9/L
Sodium	133 mmol/L
Potassium	3.4 mmol/L
Bilirubin	12 µmol/L
ALT	50 U/L
γGT	400 U/L
Cortisol	1003 nmol/L

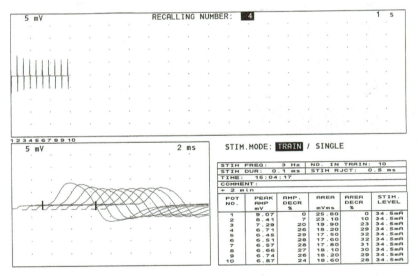

POT NO.	PEAK AMP mV	AMP. DECR %	AREA mVms	AREA DECR %	STIM. LEVEL
1	9.07	0	25.80	0	34.5mA
2	8.41	7	23.10	10	34.5mA
3	7.29	20	19.90	23	34.5mA
4	6.71	26	18.20	29	34.5mA
5	6.45	29	17.50	32	34.5mA
6	6.51	28	17.60	32	34.5mA
7	6.57	28	17.80	31	34.5mA
8	6.66	27	18.10	30	34.5mA
9	6.74	26	18.20	29	34.5mA
10	6.87	24	18.60	28	34.5mA

STIM.MODE: **TRAIN** / SINGLE

STIM FREQ: 3 Hz NO. IN TRAIN: 10
STIM DUR: 0.1 ms STIM RJCT: 0.5 ms
TIME: 15:04:17
COMMENT:
+ 2 min

1   The diagnosis is:

☐ A   Critical-illness neuropathy
☐ B   Motor neurone disease
☐ C   Myopathy
☐ D   Myasthenia gravis
☐ E   Guillain–Barré syndrome

Case 20

A 35-year-old lady gives a 2-day history of severe headache, fever and nausea. There is no history of associated neck stiffness or photophobia. On the morning of admission she had also developed ocular pain and swelling bilaterally and diplopia.

On examination she had a temperature of 39 °C; she was alert and orientated. Her face is shown below. Pupillary responses were sluggish. Her visual acuity was 6/6 bilaterally; fundoscopy revealed dilated retinal veins and early papilloedema. She had a complete ophthalmoplegia bilaterally. Pinprick sensation was reduced over the forehead.

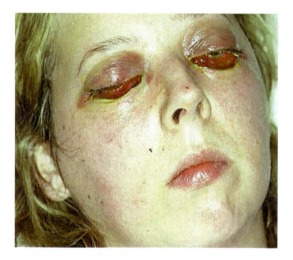

1   What is the diagnosis?

☐ A   Thyroid eye disease
☐ B   Sagittal sinus thrombosis
☐ C   Orbital cellulitis
☐ D   Cerebral abscess
☐ E   Pituitary apoplexy
☐ F   Cavernous sinus thrombosis

2   Give the two most important steps in the management:

☐ A   Arterial blood gasses
☐ B   Sinus X-rays
☐ C   Subcutaneous octreotide
☐ D   CT head with contrast
☐ E   Transarterial angiogram
☐ F   Blood cultures
☐ G   Thyroid antibodies
☐ H   MRI pituitary and hypothalamus
☐ I   Lumbar puncture

Chapter Three

OPHTHALMOLOGY

Case 1

Study the Goldmann visual field test below.

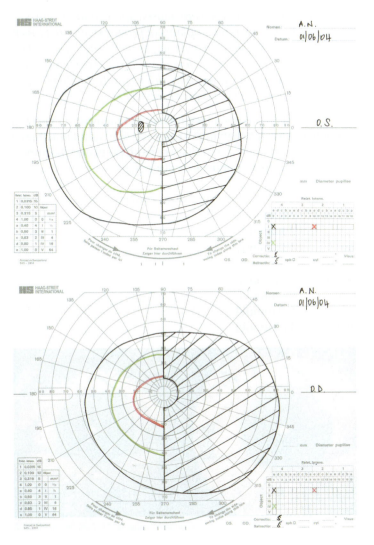

1   Where is the pathological lesion?

- ☐ A   Left occipital cortex
- ☐ B   Left temporal lobe (Meyer's loop)
- ☐ C   Right occipital cortex
- ☐ D   Right optic nerve
- ☐ E   Right parietal lobe

Case 3

A 65-year-old overweight Asian lady was referred to Ophthalmology Outpatients with general malaise and a gradual reduction in vision of 3 months' duration, affecting both eyes.

Aided Snellen visual acuity was recorded as 6/18 right eye, 6/12 left eye, both eyes improving to 6/9 with a pinhole. Dilated examination revealed bilateral, moderate nuclear sclerosis, and widespread retinal changes as shown below.

Her lipids were checked by her GP 4 months before:

Cholesterol	6 mmol/L
HDL	0.79 mmol/L
LDL	4.0 mmol/L
Fasting triglycerides	4.6 mmol/L

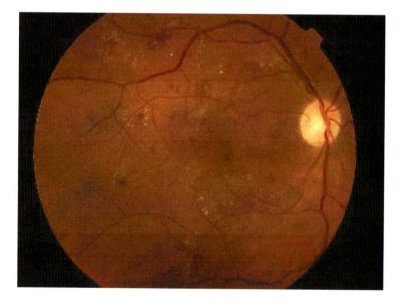

1   Which of the following is the most likely underlying diagnosis?

☐ A   Ankylosing spondylitis
☐ B   Diabetes mellitus
☐ C   Hyperlipidaemia
☐ D   Multiple sclerosis
☐ E   Sarcoidosis

Case 4

A 65-year-old man presents to A&E with reduced vision in the right eye, noticed while taking a photograph.

On examination he has a right afferent pupillary defect and the following appearance on fundoscopy

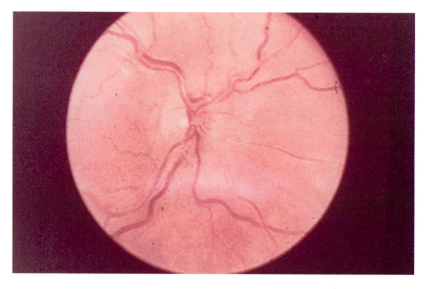

1   Which two of the following should be undertaken soon?

- [ ] A   Blood pressure measurement
- [ ] B   Thyroid function
- [ ] C   CT orbits
- [ ] D   Chest X-ray
- [ ] E   *Toxoplasma* serology
- [ ] F   Referral for fluorescein angiography
- [ ] G   Carotid Doppler
- [ ] H   Referral for intraocular pressure measurement
- [ ] I   Counsel for an HIV test
- [ ] J   MRA carotid circulation

Chapter Four

RHEUMATOLOGY

Case 1

A 52-year-old man presented with an 18-month history of malaise, anorexia, arthralgia and weight loss. He felt this was attributable to a persistent cold with a chronic dry cough and a blocked nose.

On examination he was 1.88 m tall and weighed 58 kg. He had a purpuric rash on the dorsum of his feet, extending to mid-shin. His musculoskeletal examination revealed no synovitis and was otherwise normal, except for his inability to actively dorsiflex his right foot.

Investigations showed:

HB	10.4 g/dL	Urea	3.7 mmol/L
MCV	86 fL	Creatinine	118 μmol/L
WCC	10.4×10^9/L	Antibodies:	
Platelets	497×10^9/L	Anti-proteinase-3	Positive
ESR	76 mm/h	Anti-myeloperoxidase	Negative
Sodium	137 mmol/L	Urine microscopy	Red cell casts
Potassium	4.4 mmol/L		

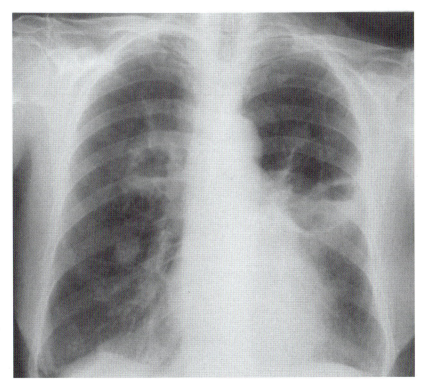

1   What is the most likely diagnosis?

- ☐   A   Wegener's granulomatosis
- ☐   B   Microscopic polyangiitis
- ☐   C   Rheumatoid arthritis
- ☐   D   Secondary lung metastases
- ☐   E   Goodpasture's syndrome

Case 2

A 44-year-old man presents with pain and swelling of the small joints of his hands with associated difficulty in gripping small objects, particularly with his dominant left hand. It has been getting gradually worse over the last 2 years. He has been feeling tired and has lost $\frac{1}{2}$ stone in weight.

Investigations requested by the GP showed:

Hb	11.6 g/dL
MCV	86 fL
WCC	10.4×10^9/L
Platelets	427×10^9/L
ESR	84 mm/ h

Antibodies:

Rheumatoid factor	Positive, 1/80
ANA	Negative

His hand X-rays are shown below:

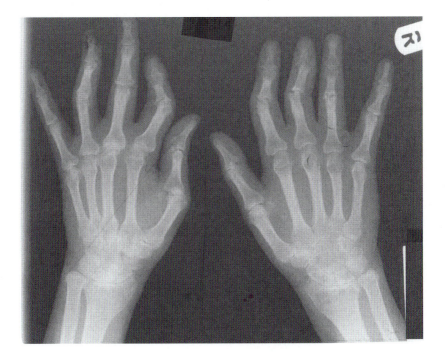

1 What is the most likely diagnosis?

- [ ] A Osteoarthritis
- [ ] B Rheumatoid arthritis
- [ ] C Psoriatic arthritis
- [ ] D Gout
- [ ] E Polyarticular septic arthritis

Case 3

A 19-year-old accounts clerk presented with pain in her left knee and ankle. She had failed to gain weight since the age of 14. She also suffered from frequent aphthous ulcers.

Her investigations show:

Hb	12.7 g/dL
WCC	5.0×10^9/L
Platelets	337×10^9/L
U&Es	Normal
Corrected Ca^{2+}	3.1 mmol/L
Phosphate	0.6 mmol/L
ALP	942 U/L
Ferritin	4 µg/L
B_{12}	100 ng/L
Red cell folate	103 µg/L
PTH	50 pmol/L

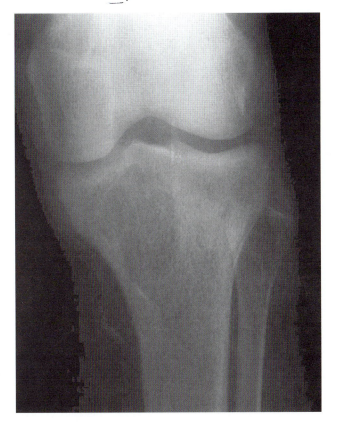

1 What is the diagnosis?

- ☐ A Whipple's disease
- ☐ B Coeliac disease
- ☐ C Localised osteoporosis
- ☐ D Enteropathic arthritis
- ☐ E Primary hyperparathyroidism

Case 4

A 42-year-old machine operator, who has had Raynaud's phenomenon for the last 7 years, presents with an impaired grip, puffy swollen fingers and difficulty swallowing.

Extractable nuclear antibodies (ENA) are strongly positive with a centromeric pattern.

Extractable antinuclear antibodies are as follows:

Topoisomerase 1 (Scl-70)	Negative
Centromere	Positive
Jo1	Negative
U1-RNP	Negative

1   What is the most likely diagnosis?

☐   A   Hand-arm vibration syndrome
☐   B   Limited cutaneous systemic sclerosis
☐   C   Diffuse cutaneous systemic sclerosis
☐   D   Systemic lupus erythematosus (SLE)
☐   E   Mixed connective tissue disease

Case 16

A 65-year-old woman presented with right shoulder pain. She described it as a deep, aching pain, radiating to the neck, with associated stiffness. The pain was worse with any shoulder movement, and worse in bed at night. Her only other musculoskeletal symptom was of thoracic back pain.

On examination she had a restricted range of right shoulder movement in all planes, with active and passive abduction to only 60°. She was also found to have fixed flexion deformities of all her fingers, though no impairment of hand function.

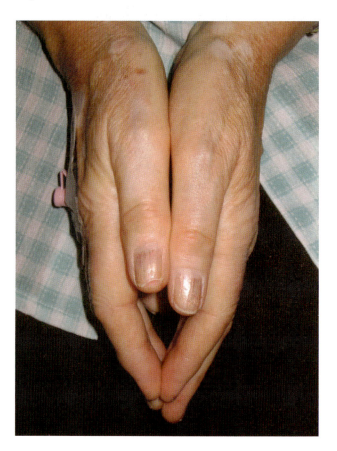

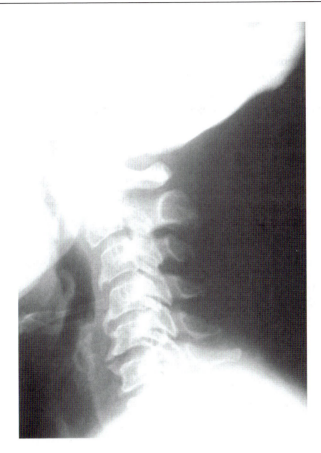

1 What is the unifying diagnosis?

- ☐ A Ankylosing spondylitis
- ☐ B Diabetes mellitus
- ☐ C Cervical spondylosis
- ☐ D Limited cutaneous systemic sclerosis
- ☐ E Adhesive capsulitis

Case 19

A 64-year-old woman with rheumatoid arthritis (RA) presented with a 6-month history of tingling in her right hand that was worse in bed at night. She had noticed that she was starting to drop objects.

On examination she had synovitis in her right middle PIP joint and her right wrist, with mild ulnar deviation at the MCPs in both hands. The thenar and hypothenar eminences in both hands were symmetrical, though slightly wasted. She had altered sensation in the thumb, index and middle finger on the right only. There was weakness of the abductor pollicis brevis and opponens pollicis on that side. Her neck movements were reduced by about 50%. The remainder of her neurological examination was normal.

1   What is the most likely diagnosis?

- [ ] A   Carpal tunnel syndrome
- [ ] B   Syringomyelia
- [ ] C   Active rheumatoid arthritis
- [ ] D   C6 radiculopathy
- [ ] E   Motor neurone disease

Case 20

A 29-year-old woman attended A&E following a fall onto an outstretched hand. She sustained an undisplaced wrist fracture that was treated by immobilisation in a cast. Shortly after removal of the cast, she developed a severe pain in that limb, worse with dependency.

On examination the limb was warm, red and oedematous. It was diffusely tender with allodynia. It was not possible to assess muscle strength due to the pain.

1   What is the most likely diagnosis?

- [ ] A   Axillary vein thrombosis
- [ ] B   Cellulitis
- [ ] C   Carpal tunnel syndrome
- [ ] D   Complex regional pain syndrome type I
- [ ] E   Osteomyelitis

Case 23

You have seen a 68-year-old man who presented with pain and swelling in his right knee.

Investigations show:

WCC	14.6×10^9/L
ESR	52 mm/h
Corrected Ca^{2+}	2.40 mmol/L
Phosphate	1.2 mmol/L
ALP	120 U/L
Uric acid	0.48 mmol/L
Cholesterol	6.8 mmol/L
Joint aspiration	Cloudy yellow fluid, low viscosity

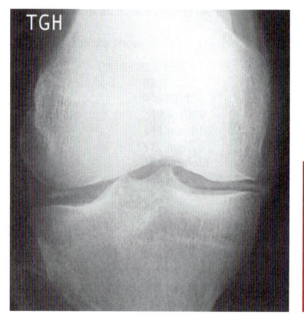

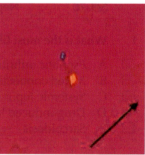

1   What is the most likely diagnosis?

- A   Osteoarthritis
- B   Basic calcium phosphate arthropathy
- C   Gout
- D   Calcium pyrophosphate dihydrate deposition disease
- E   Cholesterol emboli

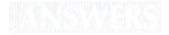

Priapism in CML is due to leucostasis in the corpora cavernosa.

2   D   t(9;22)

In 95% of cases of CML there is a reciprocal translocation between chromosomes 9 and 22. The Philadelphia chromosome is a chromosome 22, from which the long arm is deleted (see diagram). This results in production of a chimeric gene called *BCR-ABL* which defines CML.

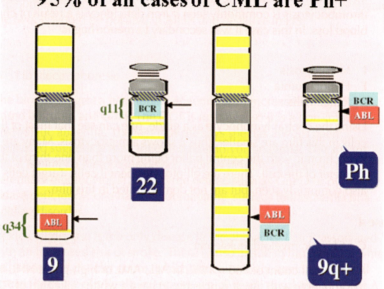

95% of all cases of CML are Ph+

Case 5

1   B   Fungal infection (typically *Aspergillus*)

The patient is pancytopenic as a result of chemotherapy given prior to the administration of his sibling's pluripotent stem cells. The conditioning chemotherapy ablates the patient's own marrow, removing any residual leukaemia, and makes room for the donor pluripotent stem cells; these engraft in the patient's bone marrow and divide to repopulate the marrow and produce the patient's white cells, red cells and platelets. During this phase the patient is neutropenic for 2–4 weeks. At this time they remain isolated, often in rooms with high-efficiency particulate air (HEPA) filtration to reduce infection exposure and are on prophylactic antibacterials (ciprofloxacin), antivirals (aciclovir) and antifungals (fluconazole or itraconazole).

The prolonged neutropenia puts bone marrow transplant patients at risk of fungal infections, which can be ubiquitous. This presentation of high fevers, pleuritic chest pain and haemoptysis and a CXR showing a circular opacity in the right upper lobe is entirely consistent with *Aspergillus*. The other diagnoses that should be considered are a *Staphylococcus aureus* abscess, hospital-acquired pneumonia and tuberculosis (check BCG scar/ethnicity/past history). The CXR is not typical of PCP, which usually shows bilateral hazy consolidation, maximal in the mid- and lower zones. The CXR in CMV or RSV pneumonitis tends to show bilateral diffuse interstitial changes. Hospital-acquired pneumonias tend to be Gram-negative – *Klebsiella*, *Pseudomonas* and coliforms can be seen. In immunocompromised patients there is often focal consolidation. TB is usually secondary to reactivation of old disease so look for old calcification in the upper zones. If there is a past history of TB, the patient will be put on isoniazid prophylaxis at the time of the transplant until count recovery.

The patient was started on broad-spectrum antibiotics (eg ceftazidime or tazobactam and gentamicin) because a Gram-negative infection cannot be excluded, but with the above history and radiological findings an antifungal should be commenced. This would be amphotericin B, the liposomal formulation if there is any evidence of renal impairment. This would be continued for at least 6 weeks. The diagnosis is confirmed by high-resolution CT. There are specific radiological features which are suggestive of a fungal infection – nodules and spiculated lesions as seen in the CT, a halo sign due to surrounding oedema and a crescent sign due to cavitation within the fungal lesion. Very rarely, the *Aspergillus* species can be isolated on bronchoscopy. Sensitivities can be carried out if the fungal species can be isolated. Definitive diagnosis is usually by CT-guided biopsy if feasible. The platelet count should be at least 50×10^9/L for this procedure.

Case 6

1   **F**   Haemolysis

The bloods show a reticulocytosis, a raised unconjugated bilirubin and LDH and a strongly positive DCT with IgG and complement. The film shows polychromasia and spherocytes. Hypersplenism will also be contributing to the anaemia by red cell pooling. This will be causing the mild leucopenia and thrombocytopenia. The iron studies – low/normal iron, low TIBC and low transferrin saturations – are consistent with the anaemia of chronic disease which will also be contributing. A production problem due to heavy bone marrow infiltration is unlikely due to the reticulocytosis.

2   **A**   Lymphoproliferative disorder
     B   Chronic liver disease (with portal hypertension)
     G   Myelofibrosis

The above three diagnoses could cause this degree of splenomegaly and hypersplenism. In chronic liver disease one should expect to see peripheral stigmata of disease on examination. Autoimmune haemolysis alone would not give this degree of splenomegaly. The history is too long for acute myeloid leukaemia and this degree of splenomegaly would be unusual. Autoimmune haemolysis is most likely to be associated with a lymphoproliferative disorder as is the paraprotein.

NB After infective causes of hepatosplenomegaly had been excluded in this gentleman, he was diagnosed with a rare T-lymphoproliferative disorder which is associated with rheumatoid arthritis, by demonstrating a T-cell clone by polymerase chain reaction (PCR) in the bone marrow and splenic tissue after splenectomy.

Case 7

1   **I**   Thymoma
     K   Thyroid tumour
     E   Teratoma
     A   Hodgkin's disease
     B   Mediastinal non-Hodgkin's lymphoma

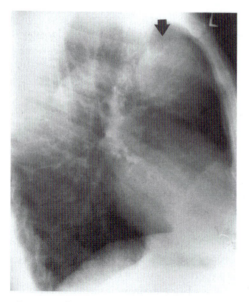

The CXR shows an anterior mediastinal mass. This is suggested by the presence of the silhouette of the descending aorta.

A CT chest will delineate the anatomy and associations of the mass and demonstrate other lymphadenopathy. An abdominopelvic CT scan should also be performed, looking for significant lymphadenopathy elsewhere; if it were to be present the diagnosis would almost certainly be lymphoma and the scan will stage the disease. If there is no better/safer target to biopsy, the mediastinal mass will have to be approached via mediastinoscopy.

All these patients should be assessed for superior vena cava obstruction, the symptoms of which are dyspnoea, orthopnoea, paroxysmal nocturnal dyspnoea, facial and neck swelling, headache, and cough; the signs are facial oedema, neck vein distension, tachypnoea and collaterals on the thorax.

2   **D** Red cell aplasia

She has a normocytic anaemia with normal haematinics and a reticulocytopenia. This suggests a production problem. The absence of reticulocytes is consistent with a diagnosis of acquired red cell aplasia. Parvovirus infection can cause a transient red cell aplasia but this is only significant in patients with a shortened red cell survival (as in haemolytic anaemias) where it can produce an acute life-threatening anaemia. It could be an immune-mediated red cell aplasia, either antibody or T cell-mediated or in association with neoplasia (thymoma, lymphoma or carcinoma).

Red cell aplasia and a mediastinal mass is suggestive of a thymoma or lymphoma.

3   **F** Tensilon® test

Double vision on reading (as the eyes tire) suggests fatigue, which is the hallmark of myasthenia gravis and in the context of a mediastinal mass and pure red cell aplasia this is suggestive of thymoma-associated myasthenia gravis. The thymoma can be benign or malignant. A Tensilon® (intravenous edrophonium) test is usually only necessary in cases where there is some diagnostic difficulty (ie negative anti-ACh receptor antibodies and an unhelpful EMG).

Case 8

1   **G** Myelofibrosis
     H Tropical splenomegaly
     E Leishmaniasis

This is massive splenomegaly: the causes are CML, myelofibrosis, malaria (and tropical splenomegaly in areas where malaria is endemic), visceral leishmaniasis and splenic lymphoma. CML is excluded as the WCC is entirely normal and the anaemia has been present for 3 years. In splenic lymphoma the splenomegaly may be associated with lymphadenopathy and/or circulating abnormal lymphocytes or it may be an isolated phenomenon. If the latter is the case the diagnosis may have to be made following splenectomy.

2 **A** Bone marrow
F Malarial antibody titres
D *Leishmania* serology

A bone marrow is diagnostic in myelofibrosis, but in many circumstances it is impossible to aspirate because of extensive fibrosis; a core of bone marrow called a 'trephine' is therefore necessary to make the diagnosis. A peripheral blood film can be highly suggestive (see below).

Tropical splenomegaly is suggested by malarial antibody titres. A polyclonal elevation of serum IgM is also commonly seen.

In leishmaniasis Giemsa-stained bone marrow smears may be diagnostic. The aspirate can also be cultured. Percutaneous splenic aspiration for staining and culture also has a high diagnostic yield but is dangerous if there is thrombocytopenia or coagulopathy. Serological tests for leishmaniasis can also be helpful.

3 **A** Tear-drop poikilocytes
I Leucoerythroblastic blood film

The diagnosis is myelofibrosis. The film shows anisocytosis and poikilocytosis (variation in size and shape of the red cells respectively). In particular, tear-drop poikilocytes are clearly seen. These occur in bone marrow fibrosis or severe dyserythropoiesis. Myelofibrosis is a myeloproliferative disorder. Early in the course of the disease there may be a leucocytosis and thrombocytosis. Later there may be a pancytopenia due to production failure as a result of extensive bone marrow fibrosis. The splenomegaly, which can be massive, is a result of extramedullary haemopoiesis. The film also shows a nucleated red cell in the bottom right-hand corner and a myelocyte, which is a myeloid precursor, in the top right-hand corner. It is therefore referred to as a 'leucoerythroblastic blood' film. These precursors are present in the peripheral blood again because of extensive bone marrow fibrosis.

Case 9

1   **F**   Sarcoidosis

The combination of bilateral hilar lymphadenopathy, a papular rash, lung disease with non-caseating granulomas on biopsy, and a lymphocytosis on BAL are highly suggestive of sarcoidosis. Acute sarcoidosis can present with a symmetrical polyarthropathy. The main differential diagnoses are tuberculosis and lymphoma; both of these diseases can cause non-caseating granulomas and bilateral hilar lymphadenopathy. The diagnosis of sarcoidosis is favoured by the multisystem presentation with skin and joint involvement. The lack of a fever goes against tuberculosis.

2   **C**   Secondary polycythaemia

As a result of chronic hypoxia, over time this gentleman has developed a secondary polycythaemia. His haemoglobin at presentation was 15.3 g/dL and now has increased to 18.2 g/gL as a result of hypoxia driving bone marrow erythropoiesis. He went on to have a radio-labelled red cell mass study which confirmed a true polycythaemia. An apparent polycythaemia occurs when the red cell mass is in the normal range but the plasma volume is decreased, giving the appearance of a polycythaemia (for example in dehydration). The treatment of secondary polycythaemia is dependent on symptoms such as headaches and dizziness. Venesection is performed if there are symptoms or if the haematocrit is repeatedly more than 0.55. Venesection would aim to bring the haematocrit into the normal range (<0.52 in men and <0.47 in women). Studies have shown that a reduction in the haematocrit leads to an increase in exercise tolerance. Oxygen therapy is also effective and improves prognosis.

Case 10

1   **G**   Acute myeloid leukaemia
    E   Myelodysplasia
    H   Hairy cell leukaemia

The blood results show a pancytopenia with the platelets and white cells being most severely affected. The anaemia is normocytic and there is a reticulocytopenia (absolute count reduced, % lower limit of normal because of the reduction in the total red cell count) suggesting a production problem. The three diagnoses in the list that can cause this degree of pancytopenia are:

• Acute myeloid leukaemia – the normal bone marrow is replaced

119

almost completely with leukaemic blasts which eventually spill out into the peripheral blood, leading to a raised white cell count, if no treatment is given.

- Myelodysplasia – an acquired bone marrow failure disorder affecting all three cell lines, commoner in the elderly. Genetic defects occur within multipotent stem cells, which lead to ineffective haemopoiesis due to excess apoptosis and therefore peripheral cytopenias. It is a pre-leukaemic condition, although death may occur prior to transformation to AML. This condition is often but not always associated with a macrocytic anaemia.
- Hairy cell leukaemia – this is characterised by a pancytopenia. This is a result of reduced bone marrow production due to infiltration by the leukaemia and hypersplenism. Splenomegaly is seen in 60% of cases and can be moderate. Patients are commonly neutropenic but a big clue to the diagnosis is a monocytopenia. Circulating hairy cells can sometimes be seen on the peripheral film (B lymphocytes with an irregular or hairy cytoplasmic outline).

2   **A**   Acute myeloid leukaemia
     F   Malaria falciparum

The first picture shows falciparum ring forms (delicate rings with double dots) within the red cells to the right of the centre of the field and in the bottom right-hand corner of the field. The second picture shows leukaemic blasts in a circle with one myelocyte at 1 o'clock. The blasts are large cells with very little cytoplasm, with an open, lacy chromatin pattern and some of them have clear nucleoli.

Chronic lymphocytic leukaemia and non-Hodgkin's lymphoma are excluded as there is no excess of lymphocytes in either field. No hairy cells are seen, the appearance of which is described above.

Case 11

1   **E**   Malaria film
     G   Blood cultures
     A   Group and save

He has just returned from a malaria region and is pyrexial. Malaria has a higher mortality in patients with homozygous sickle cell disease than in normal individuals.

Blood cultures should be done in all pyrexial patients with sickle cell disease prior to commencing antibiotics because of the increased risk of septicaemia with encapsulated bacteria and increasing resistance to antimicrobials.

A group and save should be done immediately because he obviously has phenotypically severe sickle cell disease and has required ITU admission on two occasions. The blood transfusion laboratory should also be informed of his admission if he is likely to require a blood transfusion, as he will require sickle-negative blood which is specially matched to his red cell antigens to prevent antibody formation. This type of blood may need to be ordered from the blood service.

The macrocytosis is due to the hydroxycarbamide (hydroxyurea) therapy, not B_{12} or folate deficiency. It can be used to monitor compliance with the drug. Hydroxycarbamide is an anti-sickling agent. One of its modes of action is to increase the HbF %, which has an anti-sickling affect.

He will require a chest X-ray, but as his chest is clear and his saturations are maintained this does not need to be done immediately.

HbS % measurements are done following an exchange transfusion as the aim is for the HbS % to be less than 30% in an adult to prevent further sickle complications.

2   **H**   None of the above

The film shows a number of target cells and some boat-shaped cells (pointed at both ends). No classical crescent-shaped cells are seen in this field. The number of sickle- or boat-shaped cells does not indicate the severity of a sickle crisis. In the centre there is a red cell containing a malaria ring form. This was found to be *Plasmodium falciparum*. He was treated with quinine.

3   **F**   G6PD levels

Prior to commencing quinine, G6PD levels should be checked in all sickle cell patients. Co-inheritance of G6PD deficiency is relatively common as there is an overlap in the geographical distributions of the two diseases, as in the heterozygous state both can protect against malaria. As quinine can cause haemolysis in G6PD-deficient individuals they should be closely observed following commencement.

Case 12

1   **D**   ATLL secondary to HTLV-1 infection

HTLV-1 infection is endemic in Japan, the Caribbean, Central and South America and Central and West Africa. 2–4% of carriers develop ATLL (a high-grade T-cell leukaemia/lymphoma) over a 70-year life span. Transmission is transplacentally (rare), via breast milk, sexually or via birth with pre-eclampsia, and thrombocytopenia are all features of the antiphospholipid syndrome. Thrombocytopenia and previous thrombosis are not features of acquired haemophilia.

Testing for a lupus anticoagulant is by a clotting-based assay, usually the dilute Russell viper venom time (DRVVT). IgM or IgG anticardiolipin antibodies (aCL) are tested for using an ELISA. Either or both can be present in the antiphospholipid syndrome. For the diagnosis to be made there must be one clinical (vascular thrombosis or pregnancy complications) and one laboratory feature – one or more of aCL or lupus anticoagulant must be present on two or more occasions at least 6 weeks apart.

Factor VIII levels can be measured to exclude an acquired factor VIII inhibitor: in the presence of such an inhibitor the factor VIII levels would be low.

Case 15

1   A   Thrombotic thrombocytopenic purpura (TTP)

The bloods show evidence of haemolysis (reticulocytosis, raised bilirubin and LDH) and there is a profound thrombocytopenia. The renal function and clotting are normal. The film shows a number of red cell fragments – most notably the fragment right in the centre of the field.

TTP consists of the pentad of fever, thrombocytopenia, microangiopathic haemolytic anaemia (MAHA), neurological abnormalities and renal involvement. The fragmentation is secondary to the microangiopathic haemolysis. Many patients do not have all five criteria but institution of therapy may be indicated. Neurological abnormalities range from headaches to convulsions to a coma.

The other conditions that can cause a MAHA picture include HUS (but the renal function is entirely normal) and HELLP syndrome – haemolysis, elevated liver function tests and low platelets – but the liver function is entirely normal. Fever rarely occurs in HELLP and may be a useful distinguishing feature.

Pre-eclampsia should be considered as proteinuria is demonstrated, but the BP is normal. This degree of thrombocytopenia would be unusual unless there was associated DIC (the clotting and fibrinogen are normal).

There is an ongoing debate about whether TTP is precipitated by pregnancy or whether the conditions occur together because pregnancy and TTP occur most frequently in the third and fourth decades of life. However, relapses have been described in subsequent pregnancy.

2   **B**   Plasma exchange

There is evidence from Canada that plasma exchange is superior to plasma infusion. However, there is still a more than 10% mortality associated with this condition and this is increased with delays in commencing plasma exchange. TTP occurs because of production of an autoantibody against the von Willebrand factor-cleaving protease (vWF-CP), which normally cleaves unusually large vWF multimers (ULvWF) into smaller functional multimers. The autoantibody leads to destruction of the vWF-CP and accumulation of ULvWF multimers, which leads to platelet aggregation and the formation of platelet microthrombi, particularly within the brain and kidneys. Acquired TTP is therefore another example of an autoimmune disorder.

Plasma exchange is the combination of plasmapheresis, which removes ULvWF multimers and autoantibodies against vWF-CP, and infusion of plasma which contains vWF-CP. All patients should be counselled about the risks of transfusion-transmitted infections prior to commencing plasma exchange, as during the course of the treatment they will have extensive donor exposure.

As the occurrence of seizures is frequent in TTP (especially in children) it is advisable to start anticonvulsants (phenytoin) prophylactically after just one seizure.

Other supportive measures which should be instigated are a blood transfusion if the patient is symptomatic, folic acid because of increased requirements due to haemolysis, hepatitis B vaccination because of blood product exposure, methylprednisolone 1 g daily for 3 days (if it is not contraindicated because of the autoimmune nature of the disease), aspirin when the platelets increase above 50×10^9, with daily plasma exchange, to reduce microvascular thrombosis.

Platelets are absolutely contraindicated in the absence of intracranial bleeding or life-threatening haemorrhage as they will exacerbate microvascular thrombosis.

Case 16

1   **A** B_{12} deficiency
     G   Myelodysplasia

The blood results show a macrocytic anaemia, a low platelet count and a low-normal white cell count. The reticulocyte % and absolute count are at the lower limit of normal but are lower than you would expect for this degree of anaemia. The DCT is negative. The bilirubin and LDH are elevated. The thyroid function is consistent with sick euthyroid or impaired adduction of the vocal cords); he is at high risk of aspiration and will need nasogastric feeding. Once the patient is stable, infected/necrotic areas should be debrided, and systemic treatment given with benzylpenicillin and botulinum antitoxin. Tissue and serum samples should be sent to Microbiology for measurement of toxin, culture of organism and bioassay.

The table below shows some common features of neuromuscular disorders and neuropathies which may present acutely. This is only a guide and there may be atypical features.

Table 1 Common features of neuromuscular disorders and neuropathies

	Guillain–Barré syndrome	Miller–Fisher variant of GBS	Botulism	Myasthenia gravis
Pattern of weakness	Ascending	Descending	Descending	Proximal, fatiguable
Eye movement disorder or ophthalmoplegia	Sometimes	Yes	Yes	Yes
Autonomic involvement	Yes	Some	Yes	No
Ataxia	No	Yes	No	No
Sensory signs	Yes	Yes	No	No
Reflexes	Usually absent	Usually absent	Normal (sometimes depressed)	Normal
CSF findings	Elevated protein	Elevated protein	Normal	Normal
Neurophysiology	Slow conduction velocity (CV)	Slow CV	Normal CV, small motor action potential (MAP)	Decrement of MAP on repetitive stimulation
Serology	*Campylobacter* (20%), anti-ganglioside antibodies	Anti-ganglioside antibodies, in particular anti-GQ1b (>90%)	*Clostridium botulinum*	Anti-acetylcholine receptor antibodies (70%)

Case 2

1   D   Add dipyridamole and simvastatin

The history of this patient is consistent with a right hemispheric transient ischaemic attack. He has vascular risk factors in that he is hypertensive and a smoker. There have been a number of trials showing that carotid endarterectomy should be considered if there is a greater than 60% stenosis in a patient who has been symptomatic in the previous 6 months. In this case the stenosis is on the correct side in relation to the patient's symptoms; however, it does not reach the threshold for surgery. The risk-benefit ratio may be altered depending on the competency of local vascular surgeons. A trial will report shortly on surgery for asymptomatic carotid artery stenosis.

This patient has had a failure on aspirin and so further antiplatelet therapy is warranted. It is very difficult to say which is the best option, either replacing aspirin by clopidogrel or adding dipyridamole.[1] Aspirin and dipyridamole has been shown to be more zeffective than aspirin alone in stroke prevention. Trials in the use of clopidogrel are ongoing. Given that the patient has carotid artery stenosis and borderline high cholesterol, a statin should also be added. A recent study has shown that 40 mg of simvastatin reduces the risk of subsequent major vascular events in high-risk patients, even if the total cholesterol is less than 5 mmol/L.[2]

[1] Antithrombotic Trialists' Collaboration. 2002. Collaborative meta-analysis of randomised trials of antiplatelet therapy for prevention of death, myocardial infarction, and stroke in high-risk patients. *BMJ*, 324, 71–86.
[2] Heart Protection Study Collaborative Group. 2002. MRC/BHF Heart Protection Study of cholesterol-lowering with simvastatin in 20,536 high-risk individuals: a randomised placebo-controlled trial. *Lancet*, 360, 7–22.

Case 3

1   A   Sagittal sinus thrombosis

Ulcerative colitis results in thrombophilia and the biochemistry results show that this patient is dehydrated. This puts the patient at risk of venous sinus thrombosis. The CT head with contrast shows a haemorrhagic infarct in the left frontal lobe with mass effect (this is a venous infarct).

NB a unilateral intracerebral haemorrhage would **not** explain the clinical signs on examination, (bilateral extensor plantars). The CT head also shows what is called 'the empty delta sign'. An arrow points to the sagittal sinus, which should be full of contrast. However, there is a dark central area which represents thrombus within the sinus.

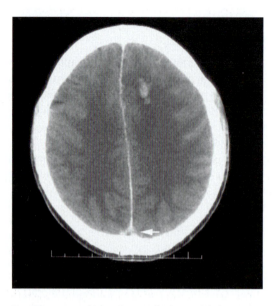

2   **B**   Therapeutic anticoagulation with heparin

The patient should be therapeutically anticoagulated with heparin. Although there is a haemorrhagic infarct, this is secondary to venous hypertension. The consequences of not treating the thrombus are likely to be dire. The patient clearly also needs fluid and electrolyte resuscitation (5% dextrose is better for *rehydration* whereas normal saline is more useful for volume replacement).

Case 4

1   **C**   Right carotid artery dissection

On examination this patient has a right Horner's syndrome. He has evidence of a right cortical deficit – sensory neglect is a cortical phenomenon arising from lesions in the parietal lobe – he also has brisk reflexes on the left. Carotid artery dissection often follows minor trauma. It is more likely to occur in patients with a collagen disorder such as Marfan's syndrome. Patients may complain of neck pain.

Regarding Horner's syndrome – the sympathetic outflow begins in the hypothalamus and then passes through the brainstem via the lateral part of the medulla. It exits via the T1 root and there is a synapse in the superior cervical ganglion. There is a complex of sympathetic nerves around the carotid artery and it is this which is damaged during carotid artery dissection. Sympathetic nerves then travel via the superior orbital fissure into the eye. This patient has therefore had a right carotid dissection; there is a high risk of thrombus formation at the site of dissection and in this case thromboembolism has occurred into the right middle cerebral artery territory.

Vertebral artery dissection normally results in a progressive brainstem syndrome. Signs will often be bilateral and one would not expect anterior circulation cortical signs such as sensory neglect.

Lateral medullary syndrome occurs following thrombosis of the posterior inferior cerebellar artery. It can produce a Horner's syndrome; there are usually associated ipsilateral cerebellar symptoms and signs, altered facial sensation and IXth and Xth cranial nerve involvement.

2   **B**   MRI brain and cervical spine

The best investigation is MRI brain and carotid arteries. The MRI cervical spine gives views of the carotid arteries and is required in particular to look for thickening and thrombus within the wall of the carotid artery. Magnetic resonance angiography may be performed in addition to show narrowing of the artery. Percutaneous angiography is not normally performed first-line due to its invasive nature.

3   **C**   Therapeutic anticoagulation with heparin

The treatment of choice is therapeutic anticoagulation with heparin to reduce the risk of further thromboembolism. He will subsequently need treatment with warfarin.

Case 5

1   **C**   Subarachnoid haemorrhage

The main differential diagnosis, clinically, is between meningitis and subarachnoid haemorrhage. The CT scan shows blood in the subarachnoid space; it can clearly be seen outlining the midbrain and in the Sylvian fissure (arrows). A large aneurysm can actually be seen in the region of the anterior communicating artery (arrowhead). In subarachnoid haemorrhage meningism is common due to meningeal irritation.

NB The patient does not have papilloedema. However, in the context of raised intracranial pressure, papilloedema can take up to 24 hours to develop. On fundoscopy, subhyaloid haemorrhages (a haemorrhage between the retina and vitreous) may be seen.

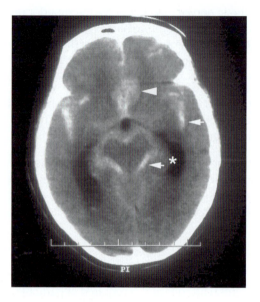

2   **B**   Hydrocephalus

Hydrocephalus has developed as shown by the markedly dilated temporal horns (asterisk). This patient needs urgent referral to the neurosurgeons for treatment. In particular, given the presence of hydrocephalus, not only does the aneurysm need treatment but ventricular shunting may also be required. The patient should be treated with nimodipine to prevent secondary vasospasm and kept well hydrated. The options for aneurysm treatment include surgery to clip the aneurysm or interventional radiology to coil the aneurysm. The choice depends on the site and size of aneurysm and clinical condition of the patient. The timing is also important as once vasospasm develops (usually at day 3) it becomes a high-risk procedure.

Case 6

1   **D**   Osteomalacia

Muscle disease often presents as a proximal weakness. Proximal weakness in the lower limbs manifests itself as difficulty rising from chairs and walking upstairs. People with proximal weakness in the upper limbs may complain of difficulty hanging out the washing or combing their hair.

Below are some causes of proximal weakness:

- Neuromuscular disorders:
  myasthenia gravis
  botulism

- Inflammatory myopathy:
  polymyositis
  dermatomyositis

- Infections of muscle:
  staphylococcus
  coxsackievirus

- Drug-induced myopathy:
  statins
  colchicine
  corticosteroids

- Muscular dystrophy:
  Duchenne muscular dystrophy
  limb-girdle muscular dystrophy

- Metabolic and endocrine disorders:
  hypocalcaemia secondary to hypoparathyroidism, vitamin D
    deficiency
  hypokalaemia
  hypomagnesaemia
  hypo- and hyperthyroidism
  Cushing's syndrome
  mitochondrial disorders.

Polymyalgia rheumatica is absent from this list, as although it can cause muscle pain it should not cause weakness. Creatine kinase (CK) is a useful marker of muscle disorders, where it is elevated. It is **not** elevated in neuromuscular disorders such as myasthenia gravis. The other conditions in this list can cause a raised CK and note that, particularly in inflammatory myopathies, some drug-induced myopathies and muscular dystrophies, it can be very high – in the thousands. Denervation of muscle, as in motor neurone disease can also result in an increased CK.

In this case, the low calcium and elevated alkaline phosphatase (from bone) point to osteomalacia. This is particularly common in Asians who have moved to the UK, due to a combination of factors, including low dietary intake and melanin in the skin decreasing vitamin D_3 formation.

The normal EEG (which is inter-ictal) does not mean that this is not epilepsy. In a significant proportion of patients with epilepsy, a single EEG will be normal and the critical diagnostic information is the history (especially if there is a witnessed account) and one ought to repeat the EEG.

Absences are usually brief episodes of loss of consciousness (lasting seconds) which may be associated with flickering of the eyelids. The patient's description of fear and anxiety may lead to confusion with panic disorder but there are too many additional features here. Patients may be more aware of their heart beating; this does not mean they are having an arrhythmia. All patients who present with loss of consciousness should have an ECG. The association of palpitations and anxiety does raise the possibility of phaeochromocytoma but this would be unlikely to give rise to an alteration in consciousness.

2   C   You advise her not to drive and that she should inform the DVLA

She is experiencing seizures and so she should not drive until she has been seizure-free for 1 year. The exception to this is if she has only had nocturnal seizures for at least 3 years. The fact that she does not lose consciousness is irrelevant. You should inform the patient that she should not drive and it is her responsibility to inform the DVLA. If one were to do that oneself, as the patient's doctor, it would constitute a breach of confidentiality.

Case 14

1   D   Spinal abscess

The patient is pyrexial, he is an intravenous drug user and he has a murmur: the underlying diagnosis is therefore infective endocarditis. Staphylococcal organisms in particular have a high risk of metastatic abscess formation, as in this case. Acute spinal cord syndromes can present with a flaccid weakness and absent reflexes and have a progressive onset. Plantar reflexes are helpful in this situation. The sensory loss points to a level approximately up to the C5 dermatome. The MRI cervical spine is a T2-weighted image (the CSF is bright). There is a bright disc at C5/6, indicating discitis (arrow); the vertebral bodies are also bright. The spinal cord is compressed at this level. Tuberculosis of the spine (Pott's disease) can give similar imaging findings but a more protracted course would be expected. An anterior spinal artery infarction can occur in infective endocarditis due to thromboembolism; the imaging findings and the involvement of the dorsal columns in this case (which have a different blood supply) would not, however, be consistent with this diagnosis.

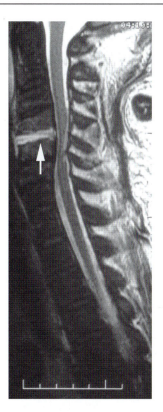

2   D   Broad-spectrum antibiotics and neurosurgical referral

This patient needs urgent neurosurgical referral for cervical cord decompression. Antibiotics (including staphylococcal cover) should also be given. It is also important to monitor respiratory function in such patients – with serial vital capacity – as the phrenic nerve is supplied by nerve roots C3, C4 and C5.

Case 15

1   E   Right ulnar, left common peroneal

2   C   Cryoglobulinaemia

This patient has mononeuritis multiplex (that is, a neuropathy picking off individual nerves), affecting the left common peroneal and right ulnar nerves.

The causes of mononeuritis multiplex are:

- Diabetes mellitus
- Systemic vasculitis/connective tissue disorders:
    polyarteritis nodosa
    Churg–Strauss syndrome
    Wegener's granulomatosis
    systemic lupus erythematosus
    rheumatoid arthritis
    Sjögren's syndrome
    cryoglobulinaemia
- Infective:
    HIV
    Lyme disease
    CMV
    leprosy – depigmented patches?
- Sarcoid
- Paraneoplastic
- Malignant infiltration of nerves.

Chronic inflammatory demyelinating neuropathy can also cause an asymmetric neuropathy. It is, however, often proximal and electrophysiology will show evidence of demyelination – reduced conduction velocity and/or conduction block.

There is a strong association between hepatitis C infection and the development of mixed cryoglobulinaemia. Cryoglobulins are immunoglobulins which reversibly precipitate in the cold (4 °C). In this case the rash, raised accelerated ESR, CRP and active urinary sediment, in combination with mononeuritis multiplex, point to a systemic vasculitic process and cryoglobulinaemia is the most likely cause. This would need to be confirmed by taking blood at 37 °C and immediately transferring it to the lab. Nerve conduction studies and EMG would also be useful in this case to confirm mononeuritis multiplex.

Case 16

1   D   Change the metoclopramide to domperidone

The patient has parkinsonism (the triad of rest tremor, rigidity and bradykinesia). The patient's history is characteristic for idiopathic Parkinson's disease. This usually has an asymmetric onset (in this case the left arm), is gradually progressive and the symptoms are responsive to levodopa. Patients with Parkinson's disease often deteriorate when admitted to hospital. This may be because they are not receiving their normal medication at the right time, or be due to intercurrent illness (especially sepsis) or drug side effects. Drugs with antidopaminergic activity, for instance neuroleptics such as haloperidol and anti-emetics such as metoclopramide, should be avoided at all costs as they can cause a marked deterioration. Domperidone is the anti-emetic of choice.

The 'Parkinson plus' syndromes demonstrate parkinsonism with additional features. The onset is often symmetrical and they respond poorly to levodopa therapy. In progressive supranuclear palsy there is a characteristic eye movement disorder of reduced vertical gaze (classically down-gaze, but up-gaze may also be affected); axial rigidity is also a feature. Multiple systems atrophy (MSA) may be associated with autonomic features such as postural hypotension and sphincteric problems (MSA-A). MSA may also be associated with cerebellar features (MSA-C). This patient was described as having a labile blood pressure and it is tempting to think of MSA. However, this is more likely to be due to fluid balance problems related to recent surgery.

Case 17

1   C   Ceftriaxone and ampicillin

The diagnosis is *Listeria monocytogenes*. This is a Gram-positive bacillus which commonly affects patients at the extremes of age and the immunosuppressed. Symptoms are usually of gradual onset. The organism has a tropism for the brain substance as well as the meninges (causing a meningoencephalitis) with particular involvement of the brainstem (rhomboencephalitis). Patients may therefore have reduced conscious level, seizures and cranial nerve palsies. CSF findings typically show a pleocytosis with a lymphocyte predominance; CSF glucose is often normal. These findings are in contrast to other forms of bacterial meningitis (most commonly *Neisseria meningitidis*, *Streptococcus pneumoniae* and *Haemophilus influenzae*) where the CSF shows raised polymorphs and a reduced glucose. In this instance Gram-positive bacilli are seen in the CSF, but a positive Gram stain is only seen in 10–40% of *Listeria* meningitis. Culture would be needed to confirm the diagnosis and this should be performed on CSF and blood. The treatment of choice is high-dose ampicillin.

Third-generation cephalosporins such as ceftriaxone are the treatment of choice for conventional suspected bacterial meningitis. They should be given as soon as the diagnosis is suspected.

Note that there has been a recent study showing that giving high-dose dexamethasone, starting with the first dose of antibiotic, in the treatment of bacterial meningitis (and in particular *Streptococcus pneumoniae*) improves prognosis. This may become accepted practice in the near future.

Case 18

1   E   Left midbrain

The photograph demonstrates that the left eye is deviated down and outwards. In combination with the left ptosis, this indicates a left IIIrd cranial nerve palsy. The association with a right hemiparesis puts the lesion in the left midbrain – Weber's syndrome. It is affecting the IIIrd nerve nucleus on the left as well as the corticospinal tract fibres before they cross in the medulla, causing a right hemiparesis. It should be noted that if the patient had a large space-occupying lesion in the cerebral hemisphere it could cause transtentorial herniation of the temporal lobe and therefore a IIIrd nerve palsy associated with a hemiparesis. However, the patient is clearly too well to be herniating.

With IIIrd nerve palsies it is important to consider pupillary involvement. The parasympathetic fibres travel on the outside of the IIIrd nerve and so are sensitive to extrinsic pressure. If the pupil is involved, (if the pupil is dilated and unreactive) then there may be a lesion in the IIIrd nerve nucleus (as in this case), or there may be a mass lesion pressing on the nerve. An important example to remember is a posterior communicating artery aneurysm that can cause a painful pupil involving a IIIrd nerve palsy. If the pupil is spared, it is more likely that there has been a microvascular event within the IIIrd nerve, for instance a mononeuropathy associated with diabetes.

Case 19

1   D   Myasthenia gravis

The figure shows a significant decrement of the motor action potential on repetitive stimulation (a decrement of greater than 15% is usually taken as significant). This indicates a defect in neuromuscular transmission and the most likely diagnosis is myasthenia gravis. The other finding one would look for on single-fibre EMG is jitter. It should be noted that some drugs, such as gentamicin, can also have effects on neuromuscular transmission. On ITU this test obviously needs to be done when the patient is not on any treatment with neuromuscular blocking agents. The first-line investigation of myasthenia gravis is to test for anti-acetylcholine receptor antibodies (positive in 70% of patients with myasthenia gravis); in a case such as this it is not feasible to wait for this result before doing neurophysiology. The Tensilon® test is now less commonly used in the diagnosis of myasthenia gravis and this is now reserved for difficult diagnostic cases (as when anti-ACh R antibody and EMG are negative). In this test, the patient is pre-loaded with atropine, edrophonium (a short-acting acetylcholinesterase inhibitor) is then given and the patient is closely observed for clinical improvement. Full resuscitation equipment needs to be available as there is a risk of bradyarrhythmia. Patients with myasthenia gravis also need a CXR in the first instance (and usually CT chest) to look for thymoma.

Case 20

1   **F**   Cavernous sinus thrombosis

The photograph shows bilateral proptosis and chemosis. An important cause of cavernous sinus thrombosis is septic thrombophlebitis often secondary to facial or sinus infections. The venous drainage of the eye is into the cavernous sinus via superior and inferior ophthalmic veins and hence thrombosis results in proptosis and chemosis secondary to raised venous pressure. This is often associated with raised intra-ocular pressure. The cranial nerves III, IV and VI as well as the ophthalmic division of V lie within the cavernous sinus and therefore involvement may cause a complete ophthalmoplegia and sensory loss in the ophthalmic division of V.

2   **D**   CT head with contrast
     F   Blood cultures

On a plain CT head the cavernous sinus may be seen as expanded and hyperdense and on administration of contrast there is poor filling of the cavernous sinus. MRI brain can provide excellent views of the cavernous sinus but may be less available in an emergency situation. Certain MRI sequences can be used to look specifically at the venous system. This patient needs to be treated with broad-spectrum antibiotics, including anaerobic cover (following blood cultures). *Staphylococcus aureus* is the most common causative organism in septic cavernous sinus thrombosis. The normal practice is to formally anticoagulate patients with heparin, providing CT head shows no evidence of haemorrhage.

Ophthalmologists should be closely involved, particularly as intraocular pressure may need to be reduced. This is a serious condition with a mortality of up to 30%.

Chapter Three   Answers

OPHTHALMOLOGY

Case 1

1   **A**   Left occipital cortex

By convention visual fields are recorded as what the patient sees. Therefore the right eye is on the right and the left eye on the left. They should be labelled to avoid confusion, but the position of the blind spots tells one which eye is which. Most other recordings of a clinical examination are recorded as if one is looking at the patient.

These fields show a homonymous hemianopia with macular sparing. The calcarine cortex, at the occipital lobe receives its blood supply from the two posterior cerebral arteries. The tip of the occipital pole, however, receives a dual blood supply via the middle cerebral artery. It is at the tip that macular vision is represented. Thus, with a stroke affecting the posterior cerebral artery (here on the left side) a homonymous hemianopia to all vision on the right occurs, but the patient will fortunately be able to read as macula vision is spared. If the same process were to occur on the right posterior cerebral artery the patient would be left with the peculiarity of 'gun barrel' fields: the patient may not be able to see a door, but can see a pin – this may arouse suspicion of hysteria in the unwary physician.

A lesion in Meyer's loop – the longer radiation that passes from the lateral geniculate nucleus into the temporal pole before passing back to the occipital cortex – affects the upper part of the field and thus the patient would have a right homonymous upper quadrantanopia. Parietal lobe lesions are the converse of this and affect vision below the level of the eye, producing a left homonymous lower quadrantanopia.

Damage to the right optic nerve would cause unilateral blindness.

Case 2

1   **B**   The findings are consistent with acute angle-closure glaucoma
     H   Acetazolamide 500 mg should be administered intravenously once
the diagnosis is confirmed

This is a classic story for acute angle-closure glaucoma. It is a disease of middle to later life. An acute uniocular attack like this is often preceded by a short period of blurred vision, often with halos round lights – particularly at night-time. Pain is a variable feature – it can be so severe and, along with the elevation in the intraocular pressure, cause nausea

148

and vomiting such that the patient is assumed to harbour gastrointestinal pathology, such as an obstruction. Acuity is reduced, the cornea appears hazy due to oedema, there is often a ciliary flush, and the pupil is fixed, often midpoint/dilated and ovoid. If the anterior chamber is viewed from the side with a torch or a slit lamp, half the iris may be seen to be in shadow and this suggests the iris is bulging forward due to the pressure in the posterior chamber resulting from the obstructed flow of aqueous – this is the shallow anterior chamber. A 'ciliary flush' refers to dilatation of the deep conjunctival and episcleral vessels adjacent and circumferential to the corneal limbus. It is best seen in natural light. It suggests either anterior uveitis or glaucoma. If suspected, it requires immediate assessment by an ophthalmologist as the optic nerve can be permanently damaged by delay.

The pressure in the both eyes must be measured, and the elevated pressure reduced. This is done with pilocarpine 2–4% drops hourly (meiosis opens the blocked closed draining angle); acetazolamide is given to stop the production of aqueous, usually orally, or intravascularly if they are vomiting (intramuscular injection is not favoured as it is alkaline and often painful). Peripheral iridectomy (either by laser or surgically) is performed once the pressures are normal – it is rarely necessary as an emergency, if medical therapy fails to control the pressure. Mydriatics must not be used as these will further increase the block at the 'closed' angle.

Conjunctivitis does not cause perilimbic (within 3 mm of the cornea) dilatation. It is usually itchy and is the only cause of a red eye that is so. It is not truly painful and neither vision, reflexes or movements are affected.

Anterior uveitis tends to cause a deep boring pain, of acute onset, photophobia (because of iris spasm), blurred vision due to precipitates in the aqueous, lacrimation, circumcorneal redness (ciliary flush), and a small pupil (again because of iris spasm) that may in time become irregular or dilate irregularly due to adhesion formation. Pus may be seen in the anterior chamber (hypopyon) with a slit lamp. It tends to affect young or middle-aged patients, and is associated with arthritides, such as Still's disease and ankylosing spondylitis.

Case 3

1   **B**   Diabetes mellitus

This is a slide of diabetic pre-proliferative retinopathy. There are extensive dot and blot haemorrhages; there are hard exudates, including a circinate exudate at 11 o'clock to the macula; cotton-wool spots are just seen, superior to the macula and superotemporal vascular arcade;

there is a large blot haemorrhage superiorly; the arteries are tortuous and fine and the veins are irregular with beading. None of this would affect acuity *per se* – in this case as evidenced by the satisfactory acuity with pinhole correction; a loss of acuity would imply maculopathy. A refractive error, or in this case lens opacity is reducing visual acuity, which subsequently improves with pinhole correction. This is difficult to appreciate from direct fundoscopy but one can sometimes get a sense that the physiological foveal pit reflex is lost, and the macula appears boggy and oedematous. Fluorescein angiography can demonstrate extensive capillary leak at the macula and show the true extent of the vascular abnormalities, including intraretinal microaneurysms (another pre-proliferative feature). Direct fundoscopy is not always entirely satisfactory at detecting retinopathy. Fluorescein angiography is the gold standard. Retinal photography should be performed for screening, and in the UK this is undertaken by opticians and optometrists. In this case, however, one should pick up the evident disease. The proximity of red disease (dots and blots) to the macula is not worrying, and can be followed up, but hard exudates (lipid-laden macrophages) and cotton-wool spots (retinal ischaemia – which stimulates new vessel formation) near the macula warrant a referral to an ophthalmologist, particularly if extensive. Any loss of acuity – even if the fundus looks normal – suggests maculopathy and warrants referral.

Ankylosing spondylitis is associated with anterior uveitis. Hypertriglycer-idaemia is associated with the appearance of lipaemia retinalis where the vessels look milky. Hypercholesterolaemia, whether combined or solitary, can rarely be associated with retinal ischaemia, but only because of proximal arterial occlusion. These lipids are in keeping with a diabetic dyslipidaemia and the triglycerides are not high enough to cause lipaemia retinalis. Multiple sclerosis causes optic neuritis. If behind the eye, this could only be appreciated as scotomas or loss of acuity and optic atrophy on fundoscopy. If at the eye, papillitis may occur where the eye is painful, with or without photophobia, and the disc looks swollen and pink. Sarcoidosis can cause a retinal vasculitis or anterior uveitis.

Case 4

1   A   Blood pressure measurement
    H   Referral for intraocular pressure measurement

The slide shows a fundus with grade 4 hypertensive retinopathy with optic disc oedema, cotton-wool spots and widespread A-V nipping. The retina looks oedematous. The other features one may see are flame-shaped retinal haemorrhages and hard exudate; which may collect around the fovea producing a 'macula star'. The presence of end-organ damage like this dictates the urgency with which this condition is managed. Obviously the blood pressure needs to be recorded and optically controlled.

This requires urgent ophthalmological assistance if there is not to be permanent damage to the optic nerve. Secondary optic atrophy with permanent visual impairment can occur.

Considering the other consequences of hypertension, the following ought to be done promptly: urinalysis, CXR and ECG ± echo to look for renal damage and LVH/strain respectively. More broadly, one must consider not only the consequences of the hypertension but also its causes, such as renal or endocrine disease.

A CXR needs to be done but not at the expense of everything here. The presence of a carotid bruit does not dictate the need to do a Doppler or MRA carotids. This is not the appearance of choroidoretinitis, which may be caused by *Toxoplasma* (which may make one think of HIV), or dysthyroid eye disease. The latter can cause optic atrophy from optic nerve compression if there is increased pressure in the orbit.

As a result of ischaemic proliferation of new vessels on the iris and in the drainage angle (rubeosisiridis) may occur thus causing a secondary glaucoma.

Chapter Four   Answers

RHEUMATOLOGY

Case 1

1   **A**   Wegener's granulomatosis

The presence of a multisystem disease with associated constitutional symptoms should prompt the consideration of vasculitis as a primary diagnosis.

Wegener's granulomatosis (WG) is a small-vessel granulomatous vasculitis affecting any organ system. It most commonly affects the upper and lower respiratory tracts and the kidney, with other systems including the eye (retro-orbital pseudotumour), the skin, the musculoskeletal system (arthralgia and myalgia more common than arthritis), the nervous system (mononeuritis multiplex) and the heart (pericarditis).

ANCA (antibody to neutrophil cytoplasmic antigens) is not a definitive test, but is often associated with vasculitis. WG is most commonly associated with c-ANCA (cytoplasmic pattern of staining, as opposed to perinuclear). The protein that the c-ANCA recognises is nearly always proteinase-3 (PR3). PR3 has a sensitivity of ~85% for WG, with a higher specificity. It is, however, also associated with other vasculitides such as microscopic polyangiitis. This diagnosis is less likely given the upper respiratory tract involvement and the presence of the cavitating pulmonary nodules.

Rheumatoid arthritis (RA) can cause mononeuritis multiplex and cavitating pulmonary nodules. It is more commonly associated with p-ANCA or atypical ANCA, when present. The diagnosis is unlikely, however, given the absence of synovitis with no evidence of chronic deformities.

Goodpasture's syndrome, like WG and systemic lupus erythematosus (SLE), can affect the lung and kidneys. It is caused by circulating anti-basement membrane antibodies. Binding of these antibodies leads to activation of the complement system with subsequent inflammation, causing glomerulonephritis and alveolar haemorrhage.

Causes of cavitation in the lung include:

- **C**arcinoma
- **A**utoimmune (rheumatoid arthritis)
- **V**ascular (pulmonary emboli, septic emboli)

- Infection (*Staphylococcis aureus*, *Klebsiella*, *Pseudomonas*, tuberculosis, hydatid disease)
- Trauma.

Case 2

1   C   Psoriatic arthritis

Radiological features of psoriatic arthritis can include a destructive erosive arthritis, sometimes with a 'pencil in cup' appearance, periosteal new bone formation, sausage-like swelling of the digits, terminal tuft resorption and ankylosis of the distal and/or proximal interphalangeal joints. The pattern of joint involvement can include the distal interphalangeal joints. There is often a polyarticular unidigit pattern, involving the metacarpophalangeal, and proximal and distal interphalangeal joints of the same finger.

Whilst the majority of psoriatic arthritis patients will be negative for rheumatoid factor, there is a small percentage that can have a low titre of rheumatoid factor. It is important to remember that a positive rheumatoid factor does not equate to a diagnosis of rheumatoid arthritis.

Case 3

1   B   Coeliac disease

The raised calcium, low phosphate and raised alkaline phosphatase generate the differential diagnosis of primary or tertiary hyperparathyroidism. A diagnosis of primary hyperparathyroidism fails to explain the low B_{12}, folate and ferritin, however.

Tertiary hyperparathyroidism is most commonly seen in end-organ renal disease and vitamin D deficiency. It can lead to X-ray bony changes such as subperiosteal bone resorption, tufting of the terminal phalanges, diffuse osteopenia, resorption of the distal clavicle and discrete lytic lesions in bone (brown tumours) as seen on this X-ray. Other rheumatic syndromes associated with hyperparathyroidism include painless proximal muscle weakness, chondrocalcinosis, arthralgias (especially of the proximal interphalangeal joints) and gout.

Whipple's disease tends to affect middle-aged white men, presenting with a migratory oligoarthritis. They then gradually develop steatorrhoea, diarrhoea and weight loss. Other features include pigmentation, lymphadenopathy and neurological involvement, dementia being the most frequent CNS symptom. Jejunal biopsies show infiltration of the lamina propria by large macrophages containing PAS+ve glycoprotein granules.

Enteropathic arthritis is an inflammatory arthritis associated with bowel disorders, commonly inflammatory bowel disease. Both Crohn's- and ulcerative colitis-associated arthritis predominantly affect the knee and ankle. In this case, the knee pain is due to the lytic lesion rather than to an arthritis. Enteropathic arthritides can also manifest as inflammatory spinal arthritis similar to ankylosing spondylitis.

Case 4

1   B   Limited cutaneous systemic sclerosis

Raynaud's phenomenon has many associations, including immune-mediated and occupation-related conditions, obstructive vascular disease and metabolic disorders; it can be drug-induced or related to infections. The strongly positive ANA in this case points towards an immune-mediated condition, making hand-arm vibration syndrome (formerly called 'vibration white finger') less likely.

The presence of dysphagia makes SLE a less likely diagnosis. The remaining three can all have dysphagia as a presenting complaint. The appearance of the Raynaud's 7 years before any other features of a connective tissue disorder, in those that develop systemic sclerosis, is more typical of the limited variety. The skin changes in diffuse cutaneous systemic sclerosis tend to develop simultaneously with the Raynaud's. The anti-centromere antibodies strongly support the diagnosis of limited cutaneous systemic sclerosis.

The symptoms of mixed connective tissue disease are commonly hand oedema, synovitis, myositis, Raynaud's and acrosclerosis/sclerodactyly, with oesophageal dysmotility in two-thirds of patients. It is associated with anti-U1-RNP antibodies. Diffuse cutaneous systemic sclerosis (DCSS) is more commonly associated with anti-topoisomerase 1 (Scl-70) antibodies.

Patterns of nuclear staining have now been largely supplanted by specific nuclear and cytoplasmic antigens. For reference, the associations are as follows:

Homogenous or diffuse – Antibodies to DNA-histone complex
Peripheral or rim – Antibodies to DNA
Speckled – Antibodies to Sm (Smith), RNP, Ro, La, Scl-70 and others
Nucleolar – Antibodies to nucleolar RNA
Centromeric – Antibodies to centromeres

Case 5

1 **E** Severe osteoporosis

Osteoporosis is classified according to the T-score as follows:

- Normal   T-score > -1
- Osteopenia   T-score $< -1, > -2.5$
- Osteoporosis   T-score < -2.5
- Severe osteoporosis T-score < -2.5 with fragility fracture

Osteomalacia is a metabolic bone disease resulting from impaired mineralisation of mature bone, most commonly secondary to vitamin D deficiency.

Bone mineral density (BMD) is commonly assessed by dual-energy X-ray absorptiometry (DEXA). The results are expressed as an absolute bone mineral density, recorded in g/cm^2, a T-score and a Z-score. These two scores are a comparison of the patient's BMD with that of reference populations. The numerical T- and Z-scores are the number of standard deviations away from the reference population mean.

The T-score represents the number of standard deviations the patient's observed BMD is from that observed in normal young women. This population is selected as it is the age group that has the maximum bone mineral density, or 'peak bone mass'. Numerically, the T-score is equivalent to:

$$\frac{\text{Observed BMD} - \text{Peak BMD}}{\text{Standard deviation of measurement}}$$

Therefore, a T-score of -2.0 means the patient is two standard deviations below normal peak bone mass. The T-score determines whether or not the patient has osteoporosis.

The Z-score represents the number of standard deviations the patient's observed BMD is from that observed in an age-matched normal population. The Z-score does not have any influence on the classification of osteoporosis. It does, however, give an indication of whether the patient's bone mineral density is appropriate for their age or whether other factors may be responsible for an unusually low bone mass.

Case 6

1 **D** Bisphosphonate

The T-score that triggers treatment is set at -1.5. Glucocorticoids increase the risk of fracture over and above the effect of low bone mineral density. Therefore, for a given bone mineral density, the risk of a fracture is higher in an individual on steroids than it is for an individual on no treatment.

Bisphosphonates have data to support their use in steroid-induced osteoporosis, but raloxifene (a selective oestrogen-receptor modulator) does not.

Recombinant PTH (teriparatide, a daily subcutaneous injection for up to 18 months) is licensed for treatment of established osteoporosis in post-menopausal women and is used in severe disease resistant to other therapies.

Evidence-based guidelines for the management of glucocorticoid-induced osteoporosis were published in 2002[1].

[1] http://www.rcplondon.ac.uk/pubs/books/glucocorticoid/glucocortConcise.pdf

Case 7

1   E   Gout

The characteristic X-ray changes with gout include bony erosions with sclerotic margins, giving a 'punched-out' appearance. In contrast to rheumatoid arthritis, the erosions are juxta-articular rather than periarticular (away from the joint line rather than at the joint itself). This gives the impression of an overhanging edge, as can be seen clearly at the left middle PIP joint. In this case, the predisposing factor to developing gout is the psoriasis: hyperuricaemia predisposes to gout. There are many states of high turnover of nucleic acid that can lead to hyperuricaemia. These include psoriasis, myeloproliferative and lymphoproliferative disorders.

The nodule palpable at the elbow represents a gouty tophus rather than a rheumatoid nodule. Olecranon bursitis is a common finding in individuals with chronic gout.

NB the presence of psoriasis and arthritis does not automatically mean psoriatic arthritis.

Case 8

1   E   Synovial fluid analysis of the right knee effusion

This patient has seropositive rheumatoid arthritis (RA) as evidenced by the chronic deformities affecting the hands, wrists and feet, in addition to the rheumatoid nodules. The history suggests that the disease was active up to 20 years ago but then entered remission. The diagnosis is a clinical one and therefore tests such as rheumatoid factor and hand and feet X-rays are not necessary.

The current problem is localised to her right knee. The differential diagnosis would be a reactivation of her inflammatory arthritis, a crystal arthropathy such as gout or pseudogout, or a septic arthritis. While she may develop osteoarthritis in her knees, possibly secondary to her inflammatory arthritis, this would not present with a hot, red, swollen joint.

Of the above differential diagnoses, the most important one to exclude is a septic arthritis, and this must always be considered when a monoarthritis occurs. Although this may lead to an elevated white cell count or positive blood cultures, neither are specific to the condition. The only way to exclude a septic arthritis with confidence is to aspirate the joint and examine the fluid by microscopy and Gram stain. Although the prime reason for aspirating the joint as the first step is to exclude septic arthritis, this fluid analysis will also be able to differentiate a crystal arthritis, and between an inflammatory and non-inflammatory arthritis.

Case 9

1   C   Methotrexate

This patient has rheumatoid arthritis (RA). This is established from the pattern of inflammatory joint involvement and supported by a strongly positive rheumatoid factor. The X-rays are normal as is often the case in early disease. Only 25% of patients in early arthritis clinics have erosions on X-ray. Erosions can develop up to 5 years after disease onset.

This patient has many features of a potential poor prognosis (young male, high titre of rheumatoid factor in early disease, large number of joints involved, high ESR, large-joint involvement, significant disability). Evidence shows that such patients should have early intervention with disease-modifying antirheumatic drugs (DMARDS) in order to prevent irreversible damage. This differs from the 'therapeutic pyramid' approach of old where patients were initially treated with anti-inflammatory drugs and only later with DMARDs.

The first-choice DMARD in early disease is debated. There are no meta-analyses of therapy in early RA. However, methotrexate is better at slowing disease progression than hydroxychloroquine in meta-analyses performed in established disease.

There is currently insufficient evidence to support the use of biological agents (TNF-α blockers) as first-line treatment. NICE guidelines state that they may only be used when two conventional DMARDs have failed, and if the disease is sufficiently active as assessed by the DAS28 score.

Case 10

1   D   Disseminated gonococcal infection (DGI)

Arthritis complicates 1–3% of gonococcal infections. Two-thirds of patients with DGI present with tenosynovitis, fevers and dermatitis. The rash may be maculopapular, vesicular or pustular. The extension of the swelling over the dorsum of the hand in this case represents tenosynovitis.

Associations between pustular skin lesions and rheumatic diseases include inflammatory bowel disease, Behçet's syndrome and Sweet's syndrome (acute febrile neutrophilic dermatosis).

The pustular lesions of Behçet's syndrome often occur at sites of minor trauma, such as needlestick pathergy. In this case, there were no other features of Behçet's syndrome.

Criteria for Behçet's syndrome are:

- Recurrent oral ulceration **plus two of**:
- Recurrent genital ulceration
- Anterior or posterior uveitis, cells in the vitreous by slit lamp examination or retinal vasculitis
- Skin lesions:
    erythema nodosum
    pseudofolliculitis
    papulopustular lesions or acneiform nodules in post adolescent patients not on steroids
- Positive pathergy test at 24–48 hours.

The rash of Lyme disease is typically erythema chronicum migrans. Arthritis is seen in 60% of infections, with about 10% of untreated patients developing a chronic Lyme arthritis.

Acute rheumatic fever typically causes erythema marginatum, with the joint involvement usually a fleeting, migratory polyarthritis affecting the large joints (knees, ankles, elbows and wrists). The cutaneous lesions characteristic of a reactive arthritis are keratoderma blennorrhagicum and circinate balanitis, with joint involvement – typically asymmetric, oligoarticular (< 5 joints) and involving the knees, ankles and/or feet. Other well-recognised features are sacroiliitis and enthesitis (inflammation at the insertion of tendons into bone).

Case 11

1   B   Spinal tuberculosis

Pott's disease (spinal tuberculosis) is characterised by destruction of the vertebral bodies and adjacent intervertebral discs by *Mycobacterium tuberculosis*. It occurs more commonly in elderly and in immunocompromised patients. The commonest site is at the thoracolumbar junction, as in this case. The X-ray shows a characteristic sharp angular 'gibbus' deformity.

Although this patient may be at risk of osteoporotic vertebral fractures from previous corticosteroid use, such fractures do not cause such pronounced angulation or spinal cord compression.

Case 12

1   A   Thyroid function

Inflammatory muscle disease is characterised by proximal muscle weakness and inflammation of skeletal muscle. This is often associated with elevated muscle enzymes (creatine kinase, AST, LDH), myopathic changes on EMG and inflammatory changes in muscle on MRI scanning. However, in this case, although the patient felt weak, there was no weakness on examination.

MRI is being used more frequently in clinical practice to locate areas of inflammatory change within muscle, allowing targeted muscle biopsies.

Proximal muscle aches, pains and/or weakness are a frequent problem. It is important to differentiate pain from weakness as a patient's description of 'weakness' may not mean reduced muscle strength.

True proximal muscle weakness can be found in inflammatory muscle disease, corticosteroid myopathy and hyperthyroidism. Other conditions presenting with proximal muscle pain include polymyalgia rheumatica (PMR), fibromyalgia and hypothyroidism. PMR is usually associated with a markedly accelerated ESR; it rarely affects patients under the age of 60. Fibromyalgia is a condition presenting with chronic, widespread pain that is classified on the presence of at least 11 out of 18 possible tender 'trigger' points.

Hypothyroidism can cause proximal muscle pain, and has been associated with large rises in creatine kinase. Other rheumatic manifestations of hypothyroidism include myxoedematous arthropathy (large-joint effusions with slow fluid waves due to high synovial fluid viscosity), carpal tunnel syndrome and crystal arthropathies.

Case 13

1   E   Polymyalgia rheumatica (PMR)

PMR rarely affects individuals under 60 years of age, and affects women twice as often as men. The clinical features include stiffness and pain in the shoulder and pelvic girdles, systemic features of debility, weight loss, tiredness, a low-grade temperature and depression, and an accelerated ESR (but not always).

There are no universally accepted diagnostic criteria, but one set requires three or more of the following:

- Age >65
- ESR >40 mm/h
- Bilateral upper arm tenderness
- Morning stiffness of >1 hour
- Onset of illness < 2 weeks
- Depression and/or weight loss.

RA remains a possibility, and can start with a polymyalgic presentation. The knee effusion could be present in both conditions. Synovitis is well described in PMR, usually affecting the knees, wrists or sternoclavicular joints. The presence of symptoms consistent with temporal arteritis, or giant cell arteritis (pain on chewing or jaw claudication) make PMR the more likely diagnosis as there is a well-recognised association between the two.

Although osteomalacia can cause pain and weakness in a similar distribution, there is nothing further to support this diagnosis, other than a marginally raised ALP. The calcium and phosphate are both normal (usually low) and there is no evidence of Looser's zones on the X-ray.

Polymyositis is unlikely given the normal creatine kinase.

Fibromyalgia is a disease of chronic widespread pain, where more than 11 out of 18 specific trigger points are tender. The absence of axial tenderness in this case makes the diagnosis unlikely, and fibromyalgia would fail to explain the high ESR and the synovitis.

Case 14

1   A   Ankylosing spondylitis

The X-ray shows fusion of the sacro-iliac joints and vertical syndesmophytes, typical of ankylosing spondylitis. Syndesmophytes represent calcification of the outer layers of the annulus fibrosis. The earliest lesions visible are Romanus lesions, or 'shiny corners', followed by 'squaring' of the vertebral bodies. The pathological changes are an initial enthesopathy (inflammation at the insertion of ligament into bone) followed by calcification along the ligament. Once these syndesmophytes meet from the vertebral body above and below an intervertebral disc, a bony bridge forms; this gives the appearance of a 'bamboo' spine.

Nocturnal and morning spinal stiffness is characteristic of inflammatory spinal disease. Decreased spinal mobility can be measured by the modified Schober's test. This measures the increase in distance between two marked points along the lumbar spine, the upper 10 cm above and the lower 5 cm below an imaginary line drawn between the dimples of Venus. The increase on forward flexion should be more than 5 mm. While an increased finger-to-floor distance may represent reduced spinal flexion, the ability to touch the toes does not exclude reduced spinal flexion as the manoeuvre can be achieved through good hip flexion despite a fused lumbar spine.

Extraspinal features of ankylosing spondylitis include:

- Peripheral **A**rthritis (large joints commonly, plus sternoclavicular, temporomandibular joints, cricoarytenoid)
- **A**ortic insufficiency
- **A**tlanto-axial subluxation with associated neurological sequelae
- **A**pical fibrosis
- **A**nterior uveitis
- Ig**A** nephropathy
- **A**myloidosis
- Osteoporosis.

Reiter's syndrome is classically described as the triad of arthritis, conjunctivitis and urethritis. It may present with low back pain and a red eye. The diagnosis is not this, however, as the radiological features of the spine differ. In Reiter's, and in other seronegative spondyloarthropathies, there can be large 'jug-handle' syndesmophytes, usually in a non-symmetrical distribution. The osteophytes of spondylosis are horizontal as opposed to the vertical syndesmophytes of ankylosing spondylitis.

Case 15

1   C   Reactive arthritis

The pain around his right foot and ankle is suggestive of an enthesitis (inflammation at the insertion of a ligament or tendon into bone). The pain in his sole, worse on weight-bearing and worse in the morning, is typical of plantar fasciitis. The pain at the back of the ankle refers to Achilles tendonitis. Enthesitis is commonly found in the seronegative

161

spondyloarthropathies, and is a frequent finding in reactive arthritis. Other typical musculoskeletal features include arthritis, usually oligoarticular and more commonly lower limb, and spondylitis.

Reactive arthritis occurs primarily in young individuals. It is a sterile inflammatory synovitis following infections, typically enteric or urogenital. The arthritis can come on around 1–4 weeks after the initial infection. Common infectious agents include *Chlamydia*, *Yersinia* and *Campylobacter*. While the arthritis is triggered by the infective process, the organisms themselves are not found within the joint.

Synovial fluid analysis can differentiate different types of arthritis. In inflammatory joint disease the cell count exceeds 1000 cells/mm^3 and in non-inflammatory arthropathies it is usually less than 1000 cells/mm^3.

Case 16

1   B   Diabetes mellitus

This patient presents with three separate conditions. Her shoulder symptoms are typical of adhesive capsulitis, or 'frozen shoulder'. This condition is usually seen in patients over 40, and it is more frequent in diabetics.

Whilst the hands may resemble those changes seen in scleroderma, systemic sclerosis would not explain the spinal features. The condition shown is diabetic cheiroarthropathy, or diabetic hand syndrome of limited joint mobility. It may be seen in up to 30–50% of long-term diabetics.

The spinal X-ray shows the diffuse idiopathic skeletal hyperostosis (DISH), also known as Forestier's disease or ankylosing hyperostosis. It is characterised by flowing calcifications along, but separated from, the anterior border of the vertebral bodies. It involves at least four adjacent vertebrae and is more commonly seen in the thoracic spine. It is also associated with diabetes, particularly type 2. Involvement of the cervical spine, as in this case, can present with dysphagia.

Case 17

1   E   Osteoarthritis (OA)

The muscle weakness in this case may make you think of a primary muscle disease such as polymyositis or dermatomyositis. However, these would not cause the firm swellings described in the question. The changes in the hand seen in dermatomyositis are Gottron's papules, an erythematous scaling rash typically over the MCPs, PIPs, DIPs and dorsum of the hand.

Rheumatoid arthritis does not have DIP joint involvement, making this diagnosis unlikely. The absence of any rash or nail changes make psoriatic arthritis equally unlikely.

OA tends to present with pain in the area of the involved joints. This is worse on activity, which differs from inflammatory arthropathies whose pain tends to ease with activity. Stiffness is a feature, particularly after prolonged periods of rest. This is sometimes referred to as 'gelling'. As pain limits joint movement, secondary muscle atrophy can occur, leading to weakness. The firm swellings at the PIP joints are Bouchard's nodes, and the single DIP swelling is a Heberden's node. The age, sex and obesity are all risk factors for osteoarthritis. Other risk factors include repetitive occupational trauma, hypermobility, cigarette smoking and a family history of OA.

Case 18

1   **A**   Osteonecrosis

Osteonecrosis is cellular death of components of bone secondary to an impaired blood supply. Common sites include the femoral and humeral heads, femoral condyles and the small bones of the hand and foot. These are sites with a limited collateral circulation.

Impaired blood flow may be secondary to mechanical alterations (such as fracture or dislocation), hypercoagulable disorders, embolic occlusion, vessel wall abnormalities, or pressure on the vessel wall. The commonest causes are idiopathic, systemic corticosteroid use and alcoholism.

In the early stages of disease, X-ray changes will be absent. The first changes may be diffuse osteopenia or a central area of radiolucency with a sclerotic border. The 'crescent' sign is a subchondral lucency indicating a subchondral pathological fracture. This is highly suggestive of osteonecrosis. Later changes include collapse of the femoral head with secondary changes of osteoarthritis.

Case 19

1   **A**   Carpal tunnel syndrome

Entrapment neuropathies occur in nearly 50% of patients with rheumatoid arthritis throughout their lifetime. Carpal tunnel syndrome is the commonest. The median nerve becomes compressed within the carpal tunnel, producing characteristic nocturnal dysaesthesias and sometimes progressing to sensory and motor loss. The median nerve supplies sensation to the palmar surface of the thumb, index and middle fingers and the radial side of the ring finger. The thenar motor branch supplies index and middle lumbricals, opponens pollicis, abductor pollicis brevis and flexor pollicis brevis (**LOAF**).

Other secondary causes of carpal tunnel syndrome include:

C **C**rystals (gout, pseudogout)
R **R**heumatoid arthritis
A **A**cromegaly, **A**myloidosis
M **M**yxoedema
P **P**regnancy
D **D**iabetes mellitus

A C6 radiculopathy can cause similar sensory changes, but would not cause motor problems in the hand. However, it is important to be aware that a 'double crush' can occur and release of a true carpal tunnel syndrome may not lead to any symptom relief if there is also a radiculopathy.

Motor neurone disease would not cause any sensory alteration.

The muscle wasting is due to active RA and consequent disuse atrophy.

Case 20

1 **D** Complex regional pain syndrome (CRPS) type I

Complex regional pain syndrome type I or reflex sympathetic dystrophy (RSD), is a collection of signs and symptoms affecting an extremity, more commonly the upper limb. It often follows a noxious, triggering event. Both limbs can sometimes be affected and, rarely, the face or trunk. If there is acute atrophy of the bones it is known as Sudeck's atrophy..

The clinical features of RSD are:

• Pain and related sensory abnormalities
• Vasomotor changes
• Sudomotor/oedema
• Motor/trophic.

The pain is severe and often of a burning nature. The affected limb is often tender with allodynia (pain resulting from a stimulus that would not normally be painful) and/or hyperalgesia (an exaggerated response to a painful stimulus). The vasomotor changes can alter with time, often being warm and red initially, becoming cool and mottled later, then cold and cyanotic. Sudomotor changes refer to increased sweating. Motor/trophic changes include weakness, muscle spasms, contractures, skin atrophy, hypertrichosis, shiny hairless skin and nail changes.

Whilst CRPS type I is often difficult to diagnose, the combination of the preceding history of trauma and immobilisation, followed by the typical changes, make this the most likely diagnosis.

Case 21

1   **D   Amyloidosis**

All of the answers would partly explain the findings in this case, but there is only one unifying diagnosis.

Amyloidosis is a disease of extracellular deposition of insoluble protein. It can be classified into the following types:

- Systemic
- Hereditary
- CNS
- Ocular
- Localised.

The systemic amyloidoses can be further subclassified into:

- A amyloidosis (chronic inflammation)
- Transthyretin
- Light chain (plasma cell disorders)
- Heavy chain and β_2-microglobulin (dialysis-related) amyloidosis.

A amyloidosis (AA) is the most common form of systemic amyloidosis worldwide. It occurs in response to chronic inflammation, be it infective or non-infective. Infections precipitating amyloidosis can include TB, leprosy and bronchiectasis; certain neoplasms can be associated, such as Hodgkin's disease, non-Hodgkin's lymphoma, renal cell carcinoma and melanoma. Of the rheumatic diseases, the three most frequently associated with amyloid are RA, juvenile idiopathic arthritis (JIA) and ankylosing spondylitis.

Sites of organ involvement include the kidney, leading to nephrotic syndrome; the liver and spleen, causing hepatosplenomegaly; and the gastrointestinal tract, causing constipation, diarrhoea and gastrointestinal bleeding.

Case 22

1   **C   Systemic lupus erythematosus (SLE)**

SLE is a multisystem disorder that can affect almost any organ system. As such, it can sometimes be very difficult to diagnose. While there are no strict diagnostic criteria, the American College of Rheumatology (ACR) have devised classification criteria for the purposes of clinical studies.

The difference between classification and diagnostic criteria means that an individual may have SLE and not fulfill the classification criteria. As an example, a patient may have a malar rash, diffuse proliferative glomerulonephritis and be strongly dsDNA-positive. This patient has SLE, though does not fulfill the **classification** criteria. That said, when SLE is considered as a potential diagnosis, the classification criteria are a very useful reference point.

The ACR criteria require four or more of the following eleven to be present:

1 Malar rash – erythema over malar eminences, sparing nasolabial folds
2 Discoid rash – erythematous raised patches, keratotic scaling and follicular plugging
3 Photosensitivity
4 Oral ulcers – oral or nasopharyngeal, usually painless
5 Arthritis – non-erosive arthritis in two or more joints
6 Serositis – pleuritis, pericarditis
7 Renal disorder – persistent proteinuria or cellular casts
8 Neurological disorder – seizures or psychosis without other cause
9 Haematological disorder:
    • haemolytic anaemia with reticulocytosis, or
    • leucopenia $<4 \times 10^9$/L on two occasions, or
    • lymphopenia $<1.5 \times 10^9$/L on two occasions, or
    • thrombocytopenia (not drug-induced)
10 Immunological disorder:
    • anti dsDNA, or
    • anti-Sm, or
    • anti-cardiolipin antibodies or lupus anticoagulant
11 Positive ANA.

Anti-nuclear antibodies (ANA) are circulating antibodies that react with antigens that are located in the cell nucleus. The interior of the cell is an immune-privileged site, explaining why all individuals do not have positive ANA. It is detected in the laboratory either by indirect immunofluorescence assays, defining autoantibodies by their pattern of binding, or by tests for specific antibodies to individual nuclear antigens using ELISA, radioimmunoassay or other techniques. These tests identify extractable nuclear antibodies (ENA). Poorly soluble nucleosomal antigens, such as dsDNA and histones, are tested using a separate technique.

A positive ANA test is not diagnostic of a rheumatic, or any other, disease. Population studies show roughly 1–5% of healthy individuals to be ANA-positive. The specificity of a positive ANA relates to its titre. The titre, expressed as 1:40 or 1/40, refers to the 'strength' of the ANA positivity. It refers to the dilution of serum at which the ANA can still be detected. A strongly positive ANA is more suggestive of a significant connective tissue disease. Fewer than 1% of healthy controls have a detectable ANA at titre $\geqslant 1:320$.

While the role of autoantibodies in connective tissue disease pathophysiology remains unclear, there are clear associations between particular antibodies and diseases:

- Anti-Ro/SS-A:
    primary Sjögren's syndrome (60–80%)
    SLE (35%) – associated with photosensitivity, subacute cutaneous lupus
- Anti-La/SS-B:
    primary Sjögren's syndrome (50%)
    SLE (15%)
- Ro + La:
    associated with congenital heart block in mothers with SLE
- Anti-U1-RNP:
    mixed connective tissue disease
- Anti-Smith (Anti-SM):
    highly specific for SLE (5–30%)
- Anti-synthetase, eg Jo-1:
    inflammatory myopathies – polymyositis (30%)
    – dermatomyositis (5%)
- Marker for interstitial lung disease in myositis
- Anti-Scl-70:
    diffuse cutaneous systemic sclerosis
    predictive of interstitial lung disease in DCSS
- dsDNA – SLE, correlation with disease activity, especially lupus nephritis.

(Percentages refer to proportion of patients with that condition who have that particular antibody.)

Case 23

1   **D**   Calcium pyrophosphate dihydrate deposition disease

Calcium pyrophosphate dihydrate (CPPD) is a calcium salt that can be deposited in cartilage-causing chondrocalcinosis on X-rays, as seen in this case. While this chondrocalcinosis can be asymptomatic, an acute crystal arthritis can be caused if CPPD crystals are released into a joint. 'Pseudogout' is the term used for this acute arthritis caused by CPPD crystals. The diagnosis is confirmed by synovial fluid analysis. CPPD crystals are typically rectangular or rhomboid and are weakly positively birefringent under polarised light microscopy. This is in contrast to the needle-shaped crystals of monosodium urate in gout, which are negatively birefringent.

Basic calcium phosphate (BCP) crystals are most commonly associated with an arthropathy at the shoulder, or Milwaukee shoulder. The destructive arthritis at the finger due to BCP crystals has been called 'Philadelphia finger'. This is a severe degenerative arthritis, often with a large joint effusion. BCP crystals are composed of calcium hydroxyapatite and other calcium-containing minerals. Aggregate BCP crystals can look like 'shiny coins' on light microscopy. They are not birefringent and therefore cannot be seen on polarised light microscopy.

Cholesterol crystals are most often seen as broad plates with a notched corner. They are found in synovial fluid, most commonly as a complication of rheumatoid arthritis.

Cholesterol emboli can occur after an invasive procedure such as coronary angiography. Clinically this often resembles vasculitis, with a purpuric rash in the lower extremities.

The numbers in this index refer to the chapter and question numbers. The topics shown may not always be in the question, but may appear in the explanatory answers.

PasTest

PasTest has been established since 1972 and is the leading provider of exam-related medical revision courses and books in the UK. The company has a dedicated customer services team to ensure that doctors can easily get up-to-date information about our products and to ensure that their orders are dealt with efficiently. Our extensive experience means that we are always one step ahead when it comes to knowledge of the current trends and contents of the Royal College exams.

PasTest revision books have helped thousands of candidates prepare for their exams. These may be purchased through bookshops, over the telephone or online at our website. All books are reviewed prior to publication to ensure that they mirror the needs of candidates and therefore act as an invaluable aid to exam preparation.

100% Money Back Guarantee
We're sure you will find our study books invaluable, but in the unlikely event that you are not entirely happy, we will give you your money back – guaranteed.

Delivery to your Door
With a busy lifestyle, nobody enjoys walking to the shops for something that may or may not be in stock. Let us take the hassle and deliver direct to your door. We will despatch your book within 24 hours of receiving your order. We also offer free delivery on books for medical students to UK addresses.

How to Order
www.pastest.co.uk
To order books safely and securely online, shop at our website.

Telephone: +44 (0)1565 752000
Have your credit card to hand when you call.
Fax: +44 (0) 1565 650264
Fax your order with your debit or credit card details.

PasTest Ltd, FREEPOST, Knutsford, Cheshire WA16 7BR
Send your order with your cheque (made payable to PasTest Ltd) and debit or credit card details to the above address. (Please complete your address details on the reverse of the cheque.)

PasTest Courses

PASTEST: the key to exam success, the key to your future

PasTest is dedicated to helping doctors to pass their professional examinations. We have 30 years of specialist experience in medical education and over 3000 doctors attend our revision courses each year.

Experienced lecturers:
Many of our lecturers are also examiners and teach in a lively and interesting way in order to:
- reflect current trends in exams
- give plenty of mock exam practice
- provide valuable advice on exam technique

Outstanding accelerated learning:
Our up-to-date and relevant course material includes MCQs, colour slides, X-rays, ECGs, EEGs, clinical cases, data interpretations, mock exams, vivas and extensive course notes which provide:
- hundreds of high quality questions with detailed answers and explanations
- succinct notes, diagrams and charts

Personal attention:
Active participation is encouraged on these courses, so in order to give personal tuition and to answer individual questions our course numbers are limited. Book early to avoid disappointment.

Choice of courses:
PasTest has developed a wide range of high quality interactive courses in different cities around the UK to suit your individual needs.

What other candidates have said about our courses:
'Absolutely brilliant – I would not have passed without it! Thank you.'
Dr Charitha Rajapakse, London.

'Excellent, enjoyable, extremely hard work but worth every penny.'
Dr Helen Binns, Oxford.

For further details contact:
PasTest Ltd, Egerton Court, Parkgate Estate
Knutsford, Cheshire WA16 8DX, UK.
Telephone: 01565 752000 Fax: 01565 650264
e-mail: courses@pastest.co.uk   web site: www.pastest.co.uk